To S

God Bless & S

Bill Goss

D0822430

About Bill's Story

"Bill Goss has written a book with a heart that keeps on beating page after page. *THE LUCKIEST UNLUCKY MAN ALIVE* is the joyous true tale of not just one miracle—but of many. It will inspire readers to live each and every day to its fullest, and most of all, to believe we are alive for a reason. The best books are those that make you laugh and cry, and, after reading them, become a part of your own life experience—this is one of them. Bill Goss will surely become an Earth Angel to anyone who picks up this book."

—Jerry and Lorin Biederman
authors, *Earth Angels: True Stories About Real People Who Bring Heaven to Earth*

"Reading *THE LUCKIEST UNLUCKY MAN ALIVE* is like going on an adventure without leaving your seat!"

—Sandra Crowe
speaker and author, *When Strangling Isn't an Option...*

"If Goss' many dances with death in the past seem miraculous, his next would be his narrowest escape ever. Just weeks after returning from an exhilarating flight [breaking the sound barrier], Lt. Commander William Goss would look closer into the face of death than ever before.... Dr. Eric Weiss of the Jacksonville Naval Hospital says Goss was facing astronomical odds.... Bill Goss is now writing a book about all his experiences called *THE LUCKIEST UNLUCKY MAN ALIVE* and there's no surprise that there's even talk of turning his story into a movie.... I would think Hollywood's biggest stars would be jumping for that one—ABSOLUTELY!!!"

—Phil Shuman/Brad Goode/Libby Weaver
EXTRA, an international celebrity TV news syndicate

"Written by the survivor of more crack-ups than Evel Knievel, *The Luckiest Unlucky Man Alive* is a work of extreme exuberance...it'll give you an old-fashioned contact high!"

—Will Blythe
literary editor, *ESQUIRE* Magazine

"He's the best almost dead guy we've ever had on the air with us!"

—Dave and Geri, Hosts
Lite Rock 95.7, Grand Rapids, Michigan

"Walk with Bill in his flight boots and soar with him above the clouds. Take an exhilarating ride through the ups and downs of his life while experiencing the tragedies and triumphs that bring to Bill the life challenges that have created a winner."

—Jetta Schantz
holder of 27 world records in aviation

"It's *Forrest Gump* meets *Jerry Maguire!* High-energy entertainment with a power-packed message for everyone!

—Jane Ellis
president, The Speakers Gallery

"Your interview on my TV show was an inspiration. None of my viewers will forget your account of the mishaps, challenges, calamities, and illnesses that you have survived but surely would have killed a lesser mortal. You have a natural stage presence, a polished way of expressing yourself, and a personal warmth that radiates to everyone who meets you. What's more, you are a thorough professional. I hope you do a lot more television."

—Dr. Stephen L. Goldstein
host, *We the People*, a Comcast TV production

"Promise me you'll call when the book is out...you are definitely an inspiration and this probably was one of the best interviews I've ever had...."

—Joe Manglass
WGNY AM/FM 103.1, New York

"The thought that kept recurring as I read your book was 'This should be a television series!' Almost every chapter has enough twists and turns to make for a television series that would keep audiences on the edge of their seats. It's obvious that you live life to the fullest...."

—Spencer P. Thorton, M.D.
Nashville

"Reflects a great humanity and love for life. It is truly an inspirational story and has the ability to not only entertain but to give hope to people who are seriously ill."

—Dale Elridge Kay
film producer, Los Angeles

"Get your vitamin shot today. Buy this book."

—Ken Vegotsky
author, speaker, *The Ultimate Power*, Canada

"Routinely striking down people of healthy lifestyles, malignant melanoma is one of the world's deadliest cancers. You must read Bill Goss' remarkable story!"

—Arthur Scott Campbell, M.D.
New Jersey

"Bill Goss is living proof that bad luck can only make us stronger. He has an amazing story which will enrich your outlook on life."

—Joe Suarez
host, *Morning Magazine*, WMRN Radio, Ohio

"After reading Bill Goss' stories about his plane crash and auto accident, I do consider him *The Luckiest Unlucky Man Alive*. But when it came to his malignant melanoma, it was not LUCK, but the manner in which he handled the problem. He did his research, had aggressive surgery, continued constant follow-up and made use of his support team—his 5Fs—Family, Friends, Faith, Focus and Fun. It is not easy to give the same advice to everyone, but this could be a good pattern to follow."

—Jay N. Weinberg
president, Corporate Angel Network, New York

"People want to hear about cancer...we're amazed at the numbers...it's the biggest killer in America."

—Larry King Live

"Bill Goss is truly inspirational!"

—Jim Watkins
host, KSQB, Santa Barbara, California

"Through Bill's book and through his work with domestic violence victims, we get a feel for his strength, his perseverance and his respect for women."

—Ellen Siler
executive director, Quigley House
a shelter for victims of domestic violence

"The book hits home with those of us who spent a lot of time in the sun. I am already beginning to pay for my many days at sea and as a teenager without a hat or sunscreen.... I must say I am much more educated about melanoma than I was before I read your book."

—Thomas E. Fleming
former destroyer Commanding Officer
Captain, U.S. Navy (Ret.)

"A high energy, interesting guest to wake up a morning show!!!"
                                                    —**Aaron Machado**
                                    host, KHBG Morning Radio, San Francisco

"Our listeners found Bill Goss' story of overcoming adversity, disaster, and death an inspirational tribute to the indomitable human spirit. Goss teaches us that no matter how heavy the burden, there is always a light at the end of the tunnel."
                                                    —**Kimberley Lode**
                                            producer, WPOP, Hartford, CT

"I feel the interview grabbed the audience—it certainly grabbed me. It gave them the inspiration to love life.... I look forward to the book."
                                                    —**Pat Frisch**
                                    host, KRNV News Four, Reno, Nevada

"Bill, you helped shape one of the most inspirational and enlightening programs I have ever done. I have interviewed thousands of guests and have rarely connected to anyone in such a short period of time. You are a special blend of human being and human spirit...."
                                                    —**Tony Trupiano**
                                            host, *The Tony Trupiano Show*
                                    a nationally syndicated morning talk show

"...a wonderfully energetic and positive project..."
                                                    —**Laurie Chittenden**
                                            editor, Simon and Schuster

"Bill Goss' story, *THE LUCKIEST UNLUCKY MAN ALIVE*, teaches us that, to truly feel lucky, you must first experience being unlucky...."
                                                    —**Kevin Baker**
                                    producer, WPYX FM *Morning Show*, New York

"What a joy to hear your story from the platform and to become your friend...."

—Sheryl Nicholson
author, international speaker and contributor to
Chicken Soup for the Woman's Soul

"Bill Goss has the awareness and insight of a true Master...and he's one guy I wouldn't want to meet in a dark alley...."

—Kirk Farber
speaker, martial arts instructor, 5th degree black belt

"If the target audience of *The Luckiest Unlucky Man Alive* is educated men and women ages 25 to 85—then you hit a BULLSEYE!"

—Dan Poor
former stuntman, direct marketing guru

"Your life story was the perfect after dinner keynote address—hilarious, entertaining, profoundly insightful and powerfully inspirational."

—James Preston, Meeting Planner
St. Joseph's Mens Club

"...your sense of humor, after all the obstacles in your life, made everyone take a look at how lucky they are...."

—The Kiwanis Club

"Bill Goss was a great guest! His life story is very compelling."

—Jimmy Barrett
host, CBS Radio, Detroit

"You won't want to put it down. Correction: You won't be *able* to put it down. It's that good!!!"

—Theo Androus
managing director, Capital City Speakers Bureau
Washington, D.C.

"...you did a wonderful job painting a picture for our listeners....
It was one of our best shows!"

—John Fulkerson
host, KIUP/KRSJ Radio, Colorado

"Bill, when my husband first noticed the sore on his toe, he immediately thought he had athlete's foot again. Pathology told us he had melanoma. He had three toes removed and all his groin lymph nodes. He started having brain seizures and in less than six weeks he lost his battle with that dreaded thing called cancer."

—Sylvia Rowell
Brunswick, Georgia

"Bill, thank you for being a guest on *The 700 Club* program. Many people were blessed by your interview...."

—Mrs. Jacqueline Mitchum-Yockey
senior guest coordinator, *The 700 Club*

"Vincent Van Gogh, Garp, Reservoir Dogs, Bill Goss, Evander Holyfield...losing a chunk of ear is an absolutely fantastic visual event just perfect for the big screen...and the big scream."

—Michael Erwin
Hollywood producer, sequel to *EASY RIDER*

"Bill, thanks for being on the show—definitely the top part of our day! Your attitude and positivity are damn infectious. Let's see the book!"

—John Keane
96 FM K-ROCK, Fort Myers, Florida

"If a cat has nine lives, Bill Goss must be a jaguar!! What an AWESOME story!"

—Rudy Ruettiger
Notre Dame football inspiration for
TriStar blockbuster movie, *RUDY*

THE LUCKIEST UNLUCKY MAN ALIVE

THE LUCKIEST UNLUCKY MAN ALIVE

A Wild Ride
Overcoming Life's Greatest Challenges—
and How You Can Too!

BILL GOSS

BookWorld Press, Inc.
Sarasota, Florida

Published by BookWorld Press, Inc.
1933 Whitfield Park Loop • Sarasota, Florida 34243
Orders 800/444-2524 • Order Fax 800/777-2525
International 941/758-8094 • International Fax 941/753-9396

Library of Congress Catalog Number 97-072027
Cover design and typography by BookWorld Press, Inc.
Cover photo by Carriage House Studio/Wardrobe by Dillard's
Manufactured in the United States of America

Author's Note: The events that take place in this book are real and verifiable. Literary license has been exercised for the sake of humor in the compression and the order of events to make the book more readable. Remember to talk with a good doctor before changing your present lifestyle. All correspondence to author must include a self-addressed stamped envelope due to the volume of mail received.

Quality Books, Inc. has catalogued this edition as follows:

Goss, William A.
    The luckiest unlucky man alive : a wild ride overcoming life's
greatest challenges—and how you can too! / William A. Goss—1st
ed.
    p. cm.
    Includes bibliographical references
    ISBN (hbk): 1-884962-17-3
    ISBN (pbk): 1-884962-12-2

    1. Goss, William A. 2. Near-death experiences.
3. United States.—Navy—Airmen—Biography. 4. Cancer—
Patients—Biography. 5. Air pilots—Biography.
I. Title.

BF1045.N4G67 1997   133.9'013
                                           QB197-40639

DEDICATION

To my parents, siblings and friends, who laugh often and hard, not because they should, but because they can. To the doctors, corpsmen, nurses and the Big Guy, who all played a part in my still being here.

To my patient, loving and spectacularly beautiful wife and guardian angel, Peggy, who continues to give my life new meaning each day. And finally, to our children, Brian and Christie, our Magnum Opus, our greatest work and my monuments to survival.

"If you have love in your life,
it can make up for many
things that are missing.
If you don't have love in your life,
no matter what else there is,
it's not enough."
—Author Unknown

CONTENTS

An oyster takes an irritant
and turns it into a pearl.
That's what I've tried to do
in this book.
Even though I'm no oyster,
I've taken some of the
irritants in my life,
including cancer, and
worked them into pearls
that I hope you'll cherish forever.

FOREWORD

RUDY, the story about my childhood dream to play football at Notre Dame, was turned into a full-feature movie in 1993. *RUDY* was a success at both the box office and as a video rental because the power of a dream excites people.

If you've seen *RUDY* then you already know my dream. Now I want to share with you Bill's dream.

As a small boy, he dreamed of flying like the hawks along the mountain ridge near his suburban New Jersey home. With flight school financially way out of reach, he instead worked as a garbage man and then later as a copper miner in Arizona.

But the dream lived on.

The Luckiest Unlucky Man Alive is a captivatingly rich chronicle of a boy becoming a man, and of that man reaching for the gold—the Navy Pilot Wings of Gold.

With one hilarious misadventure piling into another as Bill plows his way through life, his hard work finally pays off one day when his new bride pins on his Wings of Gold.

And that's when this book really takes off. A plane crash, car wrecks, cancer—what did Bill do to deserve this?

A beautiful family and wonderful friends—what did Bill do to deserve this?

You be the judge—but how you look at Bill's life—as lucky or unlucky—is a direct reflection on how you look at your own luck—and life in general. Is your glass of life half full or half empty? Are your fears moving you backward? Or are your hopes and dreams moving you forward? Do you have a "Never Say Die" attitude?

In this book, Bill shares with you unique insights on how

to re-focus your hopes and dreams toward a more meaningful, more enriching and more rewarding life. It's a treasure chest. Open it.

Read *The Luckiest Unlucky Man Alive* today. Read it right now. Not only will it make you laugh and cry, it will show you how to thrive (not just survive) when touched by crisis, adversity and change.

Even when touched by the challenge more than fifty percent of us will ultimately have to face—the cancer challenge—Bill can help show you the way.

To sum things up, I've only got one more thing to say...if a cat's got nine lives, Bill Goss must be a jaguar—what an awesome story!!!

—Rudy Ruettiger
Notre Dame football legend behind
the TriStar blockbuster movie, RUDY

Introduction

"You could be dead in six months." WHAM! Like a two-by-four right between the eyes, the words of Navy surgeon Bob Fisher sliced the air, creating a blinding white void of time and space as he waited for my reaction. He had called me in to discuss a small, harmless looking bump that had been removed from my left ear by a different doctor earlier that week.

That procedure had taken all of five minutes. The offending matter was jokingly referred to as "a nothing," a sebaceous, or to put it more crudely, a fatty cyst. As a matter of fact, it had taken my most persuasive side to convince the nice young doctor to remove it. While she was telling me that cysts often go away with time and I shouldn't worry about it, I remembered a story I'd heard about a woman—I imagine a somewhat large woman—who had a 303 pound cyst removed by surgeons in Stanford, California, two years earlier. Thank God my doctor sent my biopsy to Dr. Elie, the hospital pathologist, for evaluation.

"You could be dead in six months." The words seemed to echo in the stillness of the sterile room. Doc Fisher stared into my eyes as if to see into the soul that existed behind them. He searched for something he might learn as a doctor, as a person, about how people deal with such words. He must have been wondering how he would have taken this prognosis had he been on the receiving, rather than delivering, side.

He, like me, was a Naval officer, a lieutenant commander, a robust looking professional in his mid-thirties. Like me, he had a pretty wife whom he adored. Like me, he was the proud, involved father of a young son and daughter. But, unlike me,

Doc Fisher didn't have a "cyst" growing on his ear. He had hemmed and hawed at first. Then, to make him believe I was the macho Navy pilot I thought myself to be, I told him to give it to me straight. He did—straight through my heart.

I smelled sweat, not the smell of a hard workout, but a strong, nauseating odor I'd smelled on others before me who had received devastating news. It had always, and I really mean always, been news for the other guy, not me. This time, the sweat, the smell, was mine. I felt it burst forth on my hands, my nose, and my ears. Doc Fisher must have smelled my sweat. Perhaps he recognized it emanating from other people he had diagnosed who also had faced impending death. This time it was my body and my death.

I felt myself swooning and knew I had to think of something, anything, to pull my heart and soul up from the downward swirling spiral of negative thoughts. My nature, or as some might say, my BIG personality, had never accepted negativity and wasn't going to start now. The words that lifted me weren't much better than the ones still hanging in the air— "Well," I said to myself—"At least he said six months and not three."

And then I began to reflect on all the close calls in my past —how unlucky, and maybe stupid, I had been to get into so many bizarre situations. How lucky, and maybe not so stupid —to have extricated myself from them. I've never paid much attention to those knocks on Death's door. I've always just gone on to the next thing. This unique and humorous perspective had positively affected my attitude, my personality, and my very existence.

For a brief moment I smiled. My story could help a lot of people deal with the challenges and adversities in their own lives, I thought to myself. It could make them laugh, it could make them cry, it could give them hope, and it could educate them. My life has been such a wild ride. Maybe I've been through all these misadventures for a reason—to write one helluva good book.

"I'm a great believer in luck,
and I find the harder I work,
the luckier I get."
—Thomas Jefferson

"Even if you're on the right track,
you'll get run over if you just sit there."
—Will Rogers

PART ONE

MISADVENTURES

Before the Fall

Life is like a roller coaster: full of wild drops and curves. Since you can't get off it, you might as well sit back and enjoy the ride.

"God gives the nuts,
but he does not crack them."
—Author Unknown

CHAPTER ONE

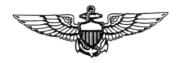

THIS CAN'T BE HAPPENING TO ME— IT'S JUST TOO STUPID!

"**T**his can't be happening to me." The thought blasted through my brain, accompanied by a series of images of my nine-year-old life.

I was watching a slide show in my mind of me and my friends, of me and my family, of me in grade school. I knew I was drowning, and this was what happens just before you go, these pictures of people and events. I didn't know it would look like a slide show.

Then, WHAM! It hit me. The last slide I saw was of my father sitting in his easy chair reading *The New York Times*. He was sadly shaking his head at the big bold headline that read—

GOSS BOY DROWNS HEADFIRST IN SINK

I can't die this way—it's just too stupid! My family would be embarrassed. It would be the ultimate humiliation. How could they explain it? What would they say? And people would laugh; I knew they would. I was drowning in a sink! I'd be dead soon, and people would laugh at the ridiculousness of it all.

You're probably wondering how anybody could drown in a sink. For me, it was easier than you'd imagine. Out of the necessity that comes from raising six kids under one roof, my dad had put in a second toilet and sink off the kitchen. It was in a closet that was so small a full size sink would never have fit—

or if it had, a person couldn't have been in the room with it. So Dad installed a tiny little sink, a lot like those in dental offices, only with faucets.

This particular day I had come home from school for lunch and had gone to wash up. I decided to wet down my hair and slick it back like Dad's or maybe Elvis Presley's. There were, after all, several of my friends and family waiting for me in the next room and I figured they'd be impressed. I filled the itsy bitsy sink with water and stuck my head in to wet my hair. Instantly, the faucets reached forward and clamped themselves to the back of my head, successfully trapping my face under the deadly pool of water. I felt it happen and knew that impressing my family and friends with tidy hair wasn't worth this. I jerked my head back—no luck. The faucets tightened on my swelling skull as if they were possessed by some demon determined to rid the world of young William A. Goss. I tried to twist my head but it was hopelessly locked and wouldn't turn in either direction. The seconds ticked by. I kicked the wall behind me, trying to get my mother's attention. My screams dissipated into gurgling noises, since my face was immersed in the water.

Unaware of what was happening to me, no one came to my rescue. But what would they have done if they had? I thought I could save myself. Time was running out—again, no luck. My head was too big and the basin too small. There was simply no way I could get my hands around my face to unplug the lifesaving stopper and drain the water. Neither could I move my face down enough to pull it out with my teeth. That's when I knew I was going to die. There was nothing I could do to save myself and no one was going to save me.

The slide show started as the oxygen in my brain depleted and I began to give up the struggle to regain the breathing world.

Innocuous little pictures clicked on and off in my mind. There were about ten of them. And then that dreadful headline, that clearly readable front-page article that told the world of my stupid death. It was more than a proud nine-year-old could stand. In a final burst of adrenaline, strength and resolve

I threw my head backward as hard as I could.

I crashed into the wall behind me nearly knocking a hole in the wall and almost rendering me unconscious. My lip was bleeding profusely—I had bitten through it—and there was a trickle of blood in my boyishly blond wet hair. The faucets had torn at me, trying to thwart my escape. Still, they had the worst of it. Those faucets were bent and bent good. Dad had to replace them.

Anyway, there I was, bleeding and hurting. The crashing noise of my escape brought my mother and friends rushing in. "What in the world have you done?" she asked. I was gagging and started to cry, then thought better of it and stopped the tears before my friends noticed. She cleaned me up, fed me lunch and sent me back to school with the others. The entire adventure—drowning, slide show, lunch and all, took less than an hour. That was my first near death experience. It was also my first important lesson about life—no matter what happens, pick yourself up, dust yourself off, and get on to the next thing.

Later, I found out that everyone had heard me in the lavatory, banging around and making noise. They thought I was intentionally making animal sounds to amuse them. Brother Larry, sister Peggy, and neighbor Chris McHugh, or "Cubie" as we called him, were all having a grand time laughing at my foolishness. Stupid noises like those were not uncommon out of my mouth. I was lucky that day, but then again, I was damn unlucky as well, all things considered. It was to be a trend in my life.

Like Dad always says, "Billy could fall into a pile of cow manure and find a diamond buried in the tread of one of his sneakers when he finally climbed out." Eugene Joseph Goss is the deep thinker in the family, making us kids think too. He's also very physical. Dad and I sparred together from the time I was old enough to put on the tiny leather boxing gloves he had bought for my brothers and me. Later, he would box me wearing the fencing mask that I had worn briefly on the school fencing team so he wouldn't have to go to work with a black eye.

"Don't ever be a bully," he'd say, "But if you're sure somebody's going to hit you—hit him first." A firm disciplinarian and loving father, he toughened me at an early age, much like his dad, a powerfully built stonecutter and sculptor of cathedral angels, had toughened him.

When my father's little sister died of pneumonia, he witnessed his normally stoic parents grieve for months. Dad watched his father, in their tiny backyard, carve an eight-foot angel from a giant piece of limestone he had painstakingly selected for her tombstone. Her death and its effect on my grandparents gave my dad an early insight into a hard world. He grew up "Down Neck," a distinctive part of Newark, New Jersey, known for its ethnic diversity, where nothing came easy and success was hard to find.

My mother, on the other hand, had a decidedly more white-collar upbringing. Barbara T. Dacey Goss, while undoubtedly as strong, intelligent and charismatic a character as my Dad, has a much more powerful sense of the "here and now." There's always been a lot of adventure and curiosity about her. I think of her as an optimizer. She taught us to always find a way to extract the very most from any situation. There are no strangers in my mother's world—none. Zero. Before she can finish a cup of coffee at a gathering of strangers she will know everyone in the room. She'll discover some familial link with each of them, even if it goes all the way back to Lucy. Oh, not our Aunt Lucy, but the Neanderthal Lucy whose three million year old remains were discovered by famed anthropologist Donald Johanson on the plains of Africa.

Mother's middle name is Tennyson, which I thought would have been difficult to handle for a girl growing up. Nana, her mom, never missed an opportunity to proclaim herself and my mother the namesakes of Sir Alfred Lord Tennyson. Although the famous poet laureate of "The Charge of the Light Brigade" was once believed to be a great, great uncle on my mother's side, I've always identified with William Shakespeare, who was born and died on my birthday, April twenty-third.

Nana had a profound effect upon my life in a very obtuse way. I was naturally left-handed and she insisted that I learn to eat and write with my right hand, saying I'd smear the wet ink and bump elbows at the dinner table if I did these things "lefty." But she didn't give a hoot which hand I used for throwing or which foot I used for kicking. So, athletically, I stayed a lefty. Nana never let up until I had successfully switched over to her school (or hand) of thought. Psychologists now discourage this sort of thing. My wife, with a background in education, believes that irreparable damage was done to my child psyche. I, however, think it forced me to use both sides of my brain more. It made my brain ambidextrous. Even my S.A.T scores were very evenly balanced between verbal and math. I owe Nana a debt of gratitude for her strong encouragement in making my left and right lobes work extra hard at getting along with each other at a critical juncture in my early childhood development.

My mother's dad, Charles Dacey, or "Pop" as we kids called him, had flown JN-4 Jennys in World War I. He was an artist, a musician, a fine woodworker and an all around handyman. The paintings and furniture he created now grace all his grandchildren's homes. Both Pop and Nana graduated from college, he with a master's degree from Rutgers. They were unusually well educated for a couple of people born in the nineteenth century. Pop, a Newark high school teacher, was always making people laugh. He was fond of telling me, "Billy, money isn't everything, but it's a reasonable facsimile."

Every summer he and Nana would have my parents and us six Gosslings up to Cape Cod, Massachusetts, for a couple of weeks. There they had put together a prefabricated cottage that the forever-innovative Pop had built in their garage in New Jersey. They flatbed-trucked it up to the Cape and placed it on a wooded lot they had purchased for two hundred dollars. On Sundays we'd sometimes see the Kennedy's in the church we went to in Hyannis Port, with John Jr. up on his father's shoulders.

I once asked Pop how he managed to do so much. "Nana

and I took advantage of everything cultural," he said, "and we weren't afraid to take chances. I decided years ago that I would accomplish something, anything, no matter how small or large, each and every day. I built the Cape house while the two fellows next door listened to Red Sox games—they're both dead now...."

After Pop graduated aviation ground school in 1917 at Princeton University, the U.S. Army Signal Corps (there was no U.S. Air Force back then) transferred him to Love Field, in Dallas. When he was in his eighties, Pop gave me his leather flying vest—from one aviator to another—to commemorate my having soloed a military training plane like he had 62 years earlier. The vest carries the faded signatures of all his long-dead pilot buddies. One was his best friend, a man whose body Pop had to return to Massachusetts in a pine box after a spin demonstration had gone fatally awry. In 1918, pilots hadn't yet figured out how to recover airplanes from a spin, pulling the stick back instead of pushing it forward to break the stall. Hell, Orville had only met Wilbur at Kitty Hawk just fifteen years earlier. No doubt about it, Pop had piloted planes before most of the world even knew planes existed. To me, he was absolutely amazing.

"Billy," Pop said, holding out the vest as if it were a precious and fragile newborn child, "I want you to have this." I could feel the tears welling up behind my eyes as I accepted his gift. I breathed in the fine, sweet leather smell as I clutched this special prize, and read and reread every one of the 75-year-old messages scrawled on its back by his long gone comrades.

Our family was blessed with two parents, who, no matter how hard things got, were committed to keeping their marriage together. Mom and Dad set a powerful example of marital commitment that provided a sense of security and stability. Even when they were yelling at each other, which was often, I always knew their love for one another would keep them together. That was a comforting thought. It was remarkable how, with all the years of yelling at one another, I never heard them utter a vulgarity or use words to demean or hurt. Bad language was not permitted in our home—loud language yes, bad language, no.

A friend once commented to me, "Bill, your parents must really love each other."

"Why is that?" I asked my buddy.

"Well, if they weren't passionately in love with each other, they certainly would have divorced by now!"

Research has indicated that marriages like that of my parents, one with lots of arguing and disagreeing, aren't destined to the divorce trash heap as it was once thought. Instead, often they're the ones most likely to last a lifetime. My mother was never afraid to speak out in our household. She was confident that my father's respect for her and for women in general was so ingrained that he would never physically lash out at her. Sexual equality reigned in their marriage and set the standard for their children to follow.

Being the fourth of six children, I shared a room with my two older brothers; at least I did until they couldn't stand my snakes anymore. With the exception of our differing opinions about the snakes, we normally got along fine. I even thought I had converted them to my herpetological way of thinking a time or two. I wouldn't have minded sharing that room indefinitely, but Larry and my big brother Bob (six-feet, two-inches, 250 pounds worth of big) moved out soon after all the baby snakes got loose. The cages were designed for big snakes, not little ones. So when the tiny babies were live-born, well, they just instinctively slithered away through the large screen mesh. After that, my brothers settled themselves into tiny alcoves in the attic. My snake collection just kept getting bigger.

At one time I had over a hundred snakes of various shapes and sizes. My brothers were always complaining that the snakes smelled bad and took up too much space. Their complaints were not well founded as I saw it. I kept the snakes clean and everyone knew our room was the best zoo in town.

My sisters were always involved in the recapture of snakes that escaped in the house, unbeknownst to my parents. Sister Peggy caught one with a laundry basket. Jackie caught one with a canister vacuum cleaner. Mimi, well she was just worthless when it came to loose snakes in the house.

I had box turtles, too, and I used to watch them mate as they crawled across the bedroom floor. A small boy can learn a lot by watching animals have sex. There were assorted other creatures that moved in and out of my life and our household— as large as raccoons and opossums, as smelly as skunks, as unpopular as bats. All were at one time or another caged in my room or in the backyard.

We all worked hard doing something, anything, to make spending money. When I wasn't working at the Arboretum (for the magnificent sum of $1.25 an hour) I was up on a mountain ridge behind our Millburn, New Jersey home in the South Mountain Reservation with my friends, Rat, Cubie and Gureenie. When we weren't catching snakes, we'd lay on our stomachs in the sweet smelling grass and watch magnificent hawks soar along under the clouds. Because it, like me, was a rare bird, the goshawk was always my favorite. As a whole, we were mesmerized by all birds of prey, envying their power, freedom and spectacular vision. We wanted to fly like them, with them. So we'd watch the soaring raptors and dream of flight and catch as many earthbound snakes as we could, which was plenty.

When we weren't hunting for serpents, we would often trap raccoons, possums, skunks and other wild animals with Havahart live animal traps, which caught them unharmed. We'd keep them for a few days in a big cage I had built behind our little garage before letting them go. Except, of course, for the big striped skunks, which we had to release immediately—although we could not resist chasing them through our neighbors' yards. We just wanted to see where they would go, and it was usually under a neighbor's porch. Routinely these skunks would do what skunks do best—to annoying young boys that is—stink up both us and the backyards of our kindly neighbors. Rat, Cubie, Gureenie and I weren't always that popular with the surrounding households, but the neighbors held their noses and their tongues, and never complained.

Sometimes, I'd wander deep into the woods alone, on a serpent hunt, in pursuit of the giant black rat snake. (It eventually was caught by Rat on his back doorstep and was almost seven feet long.) On these snake hunts, I would crawl deep into the underbrush usually emerging with a harmless milk snake or garter snake. Days later I would be covered head to toe with a deep raw rash from poison ivy. It would sometimes seal my eyes and mouth tightly shut and my mother would feed me through a straw. It hurt terribly to open my mouth or move my face. My sisters loved it because it was the only time they'd get some peace and quiet. It was great sport for my brother Larry, who would go to school with the sole intention of collecting the best new jokes from his friends. Then he would run home to tell them to me, one after another, hoping to watch me crack a smile. It was brutal. My skin would split open across my cheeks and at the corners of my mouth when the jokes became just too funny not to laugh.

Moments later, my mother would hear me screaming in pain. After blasting Larry, she'd hold me as the clear, oily smelling lymph dripped from the cracks in my face, which she dabbed with Clorox bleach to dry out. Boy, oh boy, it stung, but it sure did help. For me, while growing up, the expression "he cracked a smile" had special meaning. Hell, poison ivy covered my face during most of my preteen class photos. I was a mess.

I did all the normal things that a guy did back then in high school. Normal for a jock, that is. I wrestled, played football, tried to get past first base with the girls, the usual stuff.

One day "Jungle James" Mardis, Steve Kauffman and I borrowed some cheerleader costumes from the girls' locker room and put them on. It was a pretty ugly fit with our big backs and all. Anyway, we had a soccer player, a football player and a wrestler run out on the Millburn High School football field trying to teach the real cheerleaders a thing or two about conducting a cheer. Derry Riddle was the captain of the cheerleaders at the time and she joined right in. It ended with Steve Kauffman, who looks like actor Patrick Swayze, walking the length of the football field while standing on his hands. People walking by thought he really was a female cheerleader. We saw them stop, their jaws hitting the pavement, while this long-haired "girl" cheerleader walked all around the field on "her" hands, as casually as if walking upright. It was a riot!

Steve and I became very close friends at Millburn High when we realized we shared dual passions, girls and animals. Steve was the first person I ever knew who had a pet ferret. Named Athena, he would often take her swimming with him. Being from Short Hills, the rich side of town, he could afford to support a large menagerie of exotic snakes and lizards, unlike the backyard variety of which I was familiar.

Steve was the only one of my friends who had a swimming pool behind his parent's house, and there were always high school beauties in bikinis sunning themselves by it. As you can imagine, I loved spending time at his house.

Our family has never had that strong metropolitan New York accent like the more urban areas associated with certain "exits" of the New Jersey Turnpike, once made famous by a *Saturday Night Live* spoof:

"Heh, you from Joyszee?"

"Yeah, I'm from Joyszee!"

"What exit?"

One of my good friends, Marian Falla, a bubbly, fun loving girl, had that "Joyszee" accent. For a few years, my brothers, my friends and I worked for her dad, Emil, parking cars in the Bronx Terminal Market. On weekends it served as the overflow parking for Yankee Stadium during the big Giant and Yankee games. In our spare time we became expert marksmen with our slingshots, shooting enormous rats under the parked fruit and vegetable trucks. Anyhow, his daughter Marian and I became great buddies, and we were constantly playing pranks on each other.

One cold winter day at Millburn High School, Marian intentionally slammed into me while I was digging something out of my locker. Then, imitating a busybody, which came naturally to Marian, she exclaimed, "Now Beeelleee, what do you have in this lawka that you hafta act so secret about?" With that, she stuck her head in my locker and started nosing around.

I figured one good shove deserved another. "Marian, you want to see inside my locker, well go ahead." I pushed her head deeper into the locker.

The next thing I heard was, "BEEELLEE, help!"

"What do you mean, help? Marian, pull your fool head out of my locker, so I can get to class."

"I caaan't!"

"What do you mean you caaan't?" I echoed.

"Beeellee, I'm sereeous. What I mean when I say I caaan't is just that, I caaan't. My head is stuck in here!"

I looked over her shoulder, over the big, furry, full-length raccoon coat she was wearing. The forward coat hook was jammed deep inside her nose and the side hook was latched onto her ear. She wasn't going anywhere anytime soon.

"Marian, I'm gonna teach you once and for all not to be such a busybody," I said, laughing gleefully.

Moving to the nearest classroom, I stuck my head inside and interrupted the teacher. "Excuse me," I said politely. "There's a bear with its head stuck in a garbage can out here in the hallway!" The statement seemed too ludicrous to make up, so the entire class poured into the hall to surround this unidentified creature that was covered with a thick brown coat of hair.

"This is like Yellowstone National Park," somebody yelled.

"I needed a laugh," said the teacher.

Maid Marian, as she was known, was a girl not amused. I could tell I needed to spring this trap and spring it fast. In a few minutes, I had found the school janitor, insisting he bring his longest screwdriver with him. Over her shoulder he leaned, and finally out popped Marian's head with that coat hook still in her nose. The applause was overwhelming.

A couple of weeks after the "bear" incident, and not without profuse apologies and bootlicking, Marian agreed to go to the movies with me. When I went to pick her up, her little brother, Brian, met me at the door with a dead squirrel to feed my seven foot Haitian boa constrictor, Jacque. Little Brian could always be relied on as a source for fresh snake food. Everyone thought I spelled my snake's name JOCK, but I would correct them, after all, Jacque was a boa from French Haiti.

We now had to stop back at my house to drop off the dead squirrel. Maid Marian insisted that she hold Jacque before we go—in spite of my repeated warnings that Jacque had just had a large meal a few days before and shouldn't be jostled. Marian wouldn't take no for an answer. She took off her coat and reached roughly inside the cage and pulled out the large, thick snake.

"Gently, Marian, not so rough. Jacque's still digesting last week's meal. He shouldn't be jostled." My warnings went unheeded.

Marian was wearing a fairly low cut, loose fitting blouse that accentuated her well-endowed figure. She whipped that big snake around her neck like it was made of feathers and mockingly commented, "How do you like my boa?"

Well, by that point Jacque had had enough of the rough treatment. He dropped his long tail down the top of Marian's blouse. The look on her face changed swiftly from one of surprise to disbelief and then dismay as this disgusting sound and smell started emanating from the top of her blouse. Sure enough, what I was afraid might happen, had just happened. Inside Marian's bra, nestled between her ample breasts, now rested a load, a big, big load, of incredibly wet and stinky Haitian boa constrictor shit.

Maid Marian, suitably humbled by the plethora of early warnings given her and totally unable to wash off the stench, called it a night. I went to the movies anyway, with my buddy Boobus. He didn't smell like snake shit.

Back in the early seventies, a lot of girls thought it was sexy for a guy to have long hair. That seemed as good a reason as any for me not to cut mine. It was straight and got real light in the summer. I guess I looked like a real hippie-dippy character, even if I was pure jock through and through. I loved it. My dad called me the "Blond Apache" and my family voted me "Most Likely to be Disciplined." My friends called me Wild Willy. This was a reasonable nickname compared to some of the ones my friends got saddled with, like Rat (which was short for "Rattacrackus"), Stench a la Foof, Boobus, Cubie, Chelsea, Freebs, Jungle James, Wildman Crowley, Bloomer, Gureenie, Bad Bob, Stiff, The Grimmer, Fuzz, Dan "The Man," Grazzoo, Mo, Killer and the infamous Duvalle, to name more than a few.

My parents didn't like the long hair, but they didn't complain too much. Maybe the financial concerns of a future with six kids in college at nearly the same time were more cause for worry than the length of my hair. My father, making light of his apparent inability to not procreate unless the Church loosened its position on contraception, would often say aloud to the Pope, "You got me into this mess, now you get me out of it!" Maybe, thinking back, the combination of snakes and hair and the general recklessness of youth had made them believe I was just plain crazy. They seemed to think the best thing to do was to let me find my own way through life. So I grew my hair and took care of my snakes and lived in relative peace for several years after my first near-death experience. However, I'd end up visualizing many more humorous headlines to *The New York Times*, with one close call after another, as I plowed my way through this thing we call Life.

WHAM!
Goss Boy Swallows Wasp While Bicycling—Dies

One time I was bicycling real hard to football practice. I was the starting middle linebacker. Trying to make up the time, I peddled hard and fast down Wyoming Avenue, sucking in air as hard as I could. A fleck of yellow and black caught my eye just before I sucked it down my throat. I had half swallowed a yellow jacket wasp...alive! Trapped and angry, the little bastard stung me repeatedly on the tongue and in the windpipe. The buzzing sensation in my throat threw me into a violent coughing fit and I was finally able to cough up the little yellow demon and shoot it out of my mouth like an FA-18 Hornet being catapulted from the deck of an aircraft carrier.

An acrid taste rose in my mouth as I watched the damn thing fly away and I started to feel faint. My throat and tongue were swelling up fast, real fast, and starting to choke me. By the time I finally got to practice, I fell off my bicycle at the feet of two of my coaches, Frank Close and Matt Sellito. "Where da hell, you been, Goss?" Coach Sellito barked. "This ain't no Girl Scout singalong you're late for."

I was nearly unconscious and could hardly speak. "I swallowed a yellow jacket on the way here." I struggled with the words. "I'm sorry, I'm late."

Coaches Close and Sellito looked at me, and then at each other, mystified. After all their years of coaching they thought that they had heard it all. Finally a red-faced Sellito stammered, "Well, suit up or shower up, Goss, and make it snappy!" Don't ask me how, but I suited up. Every breath came hard at practice that day, and I remember tasting the poison from the stings for hours afterward, but somehow I made it through that day's practice. Goss kids did what they were told, and they didn't complain about it. I started to see the wisdom behind this age old expression:"The man who wins may have been counted out several times, but he didn't hear the referee."

WHAM!
Goss Boy Raises SAT Scores–After Head Injury

That winter, my luck came through again the day I took my SATs. I had an ancient Italian Lambretta motor scooter that I had bought for $35. It was not a pleasant way to travel in a blizzard. Nor was it the safest. But, I went "from the frying pan into the fire" the day my friend, Smokin' Joe McMurray, spotted me enduring the elements as he drove by in his car. Gratefully, I put the scooter in the trunk and we headed off to school again.

Despite the blinding snow, we were young, unafraid and just plain stupid. As his Volkswagen slid off the road, I saw the concrete embankment step out in front of us, stopping us instantly. My head went through his windshield, shattering glass everywhere. The next thing I saw were exploding stars, like a fireworks display, a classic sign of concussion.

I'm not sure how we got the car out, or how we got to school, but we did. I took the SAT college entrance exams that day, with a bloody bandage wrapped around my swollen skull. I did okay, considering the head injury. My mother said it wouldn't have mattered.

By my late teens I'd had three near-catastrophes. I had learned that unless you're dead, you keep moving forward. One time though, I pretended to be closer to death than I was.

Cubie and Duvalle McHugh's parents had been renting the Cedar Lake Lodge in rural Blairstown, New Jersey, for years as a rustic and inexpensive retreat out in the woods. Cubie's family (he had seven brothers and sisters) were devout Catholics, like some of the other neighborhood families, and even better athletes. Our two large, outgoing families were virtual institutions in Millburn. I'm forever indebted to them for taking me on so many trips there with their huge family. Every summer, we had a blast at that decrepit old lodge. Cubie's dad had a great sense of humor. We boys loved to play pranks on him to try to get him upset, which was practically impossible.

One day we had some particularly good luck at fooling Mr. McHugh. I was fourteen years old, and Mr. McHugh had just watched me slide off the side of a canoe that his son Cubie was paddling out into the center of the lake. As he watched me swim very quietly toward him, he suddenly saw me reach up and snatch two enormous snakes off a log between us. Climbing out of the lake toward him, I held the two wild snakes above my head as they viciously bit into both my bloodied hands and arms—and they looked for all the world like deadly cottonmouth water moccasins to poor Mr. McHugh.

When I saw the worried look on his face, I knew I had him. I fell to my side jerking like I had been envenomed and was in my final death throes. When Cubie and I started laughing, he wasn't amused. Imagine the lawsuit he must have envisioned while he thought I was dying—that is until he remembered I was a Goss. We'd never hire a lawyer.

Cubie's dad got even with us the next morning. He took us to a tiny backwoods Catholic church where he sat his sons, Marty, Cubie, Duvalle, and me in the front pew directly under the lectern. Now this wasn't a nice thing to do to the priest conducting services because it is physically impossible to expect boys who are best friends to sit together in church quietly. Of course Mr. McHugh knew that. Although we had a torturous case of the giggles we were somehow surviving, even after a serious look of admonishment from Papa McHugh. Suddenly a long, loud "PEEEEEEPP!!!" came from beneath the seat of his ten year old son Marty. It echoed loudly against the walls and stained glass windows of the church. Everyone in that tiny church heard little Marty's fart break the moist still air. That was far too much for us boys to endure. We burst into loud laughter, drawing tears as we unsuccessfully tried to restrain our outburst. We all knew we were going to be in really big trouble for this grotesque indiscretion during church. But we could not stop laughing. Mr. McHugh stared icily ahead like he didn't know us. The priest, trying to complete what I'm sure went on record as the most disrupted church sermon of all time, grew very redfaced. I'll never forget how he finished his sermon that morning—"Go in peace, to love and serve the Lord. In the name of the Father, the Son and WILL YOU BOYS SHUT THE HELL UP? Amen." We froze in terror. After church, Mr. McHugh gave us his hardest look. Then he burst out laughing. Thankfully he had a great sense of humor. I sure hope God does too.

Eventually, the McHughs let us boys assume the payment and the responsibilities for the lease of the collapsing Cedar Lake Lodge, or "The Hotel" as it was commonly referred. Some guy in Europe who was supposedly on his deathbed owned it. We persuaded him to lower the annual rent to the mighty sum of $100 a year. At age sixteen we were natural-born salesmen—and proud of it.

The Hotel had been a cathouse and speakeasy during prohibition and had long since been condemned. We started calling the hotel and its lakefront acreage "The Lake," and it was the perfect weekend retreat for ten testosterone-laden high school jocks that were best buddies. We named ourselves "The Gabers," derived from a famous old golfer named Gay Brewer. Whenever we wanted to make reference to drinking beer in front of Coach Boomer Beck, we'd simply refer to Gay Brewer. Which we slurred into "Gabe...er." Simple huh? Simply stupid. That's how we became the Gabers.

We were invincible, crazy, and stupid, and yet we were model high school boys—good students and great athletes—the kind you'd want your daughter to date. We used The Lake to test ourselves, our emerging manhood, and the world. But for the most part, we were polite and friendly. The Gabers did all the crazy things you might expect teenage boys to do and some crazier things you wouldn't. It's amazing that any of us survived.

Besides having "Sparkies," a tiny backwoods tavern nearby, The Lake had some amenities, like a double deck gazebo at the water's edge. We'd climb to the top of it with our girlfriends, dive off and swim to the other side to "show" them the waterfall. Cubie was the New Jersey State Champion pole-vaulter, so we built a pole vault pit where he could practice with another pole vaulter, the inimitable Rat O'Neil. Rat wasn't so good at it, but he tried really hard. He caught Cubie's pole for him at state tournaments. Under Rat's school yearbook photograph, Gureenie got the editor to place the caption "State Champion Pole Catcher." It really tortured Rat, but it was his own damn fault. He used to brag, "Hell, nobody, and I mean nobody, catches a pole better than me!"

One day Rat was lecturing us on the trials and tribulations of wade fishing at The Lake. As usual, it was annoying. He was annoying.

It began with Rat proudly demonstrating the latest in wade fishing techniques wearing his new (and totally unnecessary) hip boots. Fuzz, faking interest, slipped up behind him and dropped a smoke bomb down the back of those brand spanking new waist high rubber boots. Clueless as to what Fuzz had just done, Rat continued his lecture on wade fishing while Fuzz slinked back to the shoreline. We sat dumbfounded, trying not to laugh. After a full minute, we became completely convinced the smoke bomb's fuse had gone out. We were severely disappointed.

Suddenly there was a tremendously powerful but muffled "WHUMP" and massive amounts of smoke started to pour out of the top of Rat's shoulder-harnessed hip boots. Rat turned around and looked at us in horrified amazement, completely convinced that God had suddenly decided to spontaneously combust someone, and that someone was he.

Standing fifteen feet away, the Gabers laughed until we cried. A horrified Rat finally dove underwater to cure his case of hot foot and leg and body. The poor lost soul...we actually had to explain the prank to him, a most unusual circumstance for Rat, a master prankster and the true genius of mischief.

Cubie and I, along with his brothers, Tommy, Duvalle and Marty, used to climb up into the attic of that big old hotel and harass all the sleeping bats. We'd cover ourselves with old bed sheets so that any rabid bats would have a harder time effectively biting us. Then we'd beat old box spring mattresses with sticks till our ears and the super sensitive high frequency ears of the rudely awakened bats were ringing. The bats would peel off the eaves and emerge from cracks in the chimney filling the air as we squealed in delight at creating so much havoc. It would have been a pretty eerie sight for a stranger to step into—five sheet-covered figures dancing around in a dark attic full of black bats exploding out of every crevice, nook and cranny. It looked to all the world like the haunted hotel that it was reputed to be.

Although I never encountered any spooks there, the other Gabers claimed they did. Late one night while they were all asleep by the big stone fireplace, they heard the piano playing in the bar. They jumped up and ran into the darkened, trash-laden room to find nothing. They went back to bed only to hear the piano keys being banged again, this time with the sounds of all the doors in the place violently opening and closing. Terrified, they ran out dragging their sleeping bags behind them, leaving Rat alone in that place. He was still sound asleep. The following morning, Rat awoke, alone. With bleary eyes, he wandered outside and found the other eight guys in their bags on the back lawn.

"Rat, we thought you were a goner!" Fuzz and Bloomer exclaimed in unison.

"What the hell are you guys talking about?" Rat queried.

After Killer and Grimmer laid out the details of how they let him sleep all night alone with the spooks, or bogeyman, the Jersey Devil or whatever the hell it was that scared them half to death, Rat just shook his head. "All for one and one for all, I guess doesn't include Rat," he said dejectedly over his shoulder as he waddled painfully away from the men, trailing a long piece of toilet paper from the bottom of his hip boot waders.

"Do you think we pissed Rat off?" Chelsea asked somewhat quizzically.

Wild Man Crowley responded sardonically, "That little son of a bitch doesn't get pissed, he gets even."

The men collectively shuddered at the possibility. Then they rolled over and fell immediately back into a deep sleep.

WHAM!
Exploding Beans Kill Gabers

You know, as much as we male-types like to think of ourselves as complex, the truth is that humorist Dave Barry was right when he wrote, "Men Just Want To Watch Stuff Go 'BANG'." But he failed to mention how competitive it is to make the BIGGEST bang. I guess over the long run, I got to the very top of the Gabers pecking order in regard to Barry's unerringly accurate "BANG" theory of manhood. I dynamited in underground mines and built and rebuilt tremendously powerful underwater explosives. I even ended up with a qualification to drop small nuclear depth bombs (small being categorized as the size of those developed during WWII) on Soviet submarines if the need arose. However, as teenagers, Rat was the Big Bang Kahuna. Without question, in the technical and abstract world of physics, analytical chemistry, and high-yield explosives, Rat was King.

When Rat wasn't trying to impress us by letting his pet tarantula, Igor, crawl in and out of his mouth, he would be concocting a new explosive chemical compound.

One time, we innocently put a large can of baked beans in the campfire to warm up. We neglected to open the can. Rat laughed to himself. If teenage boys could have masters' degrees in neglect, Dr. Rattacrackus (a title bestowed upon him that night) most certainly earned his doctorate. To Dr. Rat, it was going to be an evening of $E = MC^2$ at our expense.

After the ensuing explosion blasted hot baked beans all over our faces, mingling second degree burns with our post-pubescent zits, I noticed a faraway look on Rat's face. As he stared into what was once a campfire, burning logs now scattered about like sperm around an egg, his zombie-like look turned into a twisted smile of euphoria. I had seen this look before. It was Rat's catatonic look of revenge. What might happen next was only limited by Rat's seemingly boundless imagination.

We rebuilt the fire, and no one noticed when Rat disappeared. It was several minutes before Grimmer asked, "Where's Rat?"

At that precise moment, Rat suddenly reappeared at the campfire's edge, and in one fluid motion, slipped a Coleman gas bottle into the raging fire, wreaking vengeance upon us all. The Gabers stared as one, momentarily frozen in fear. We watched flames gently licking the outer casing of the full butane tank that the little bastard had put into the fire. Then, like lemmings headed for the sea, we streaked away from the oncoming blast. I heard Rat's demented, demonic cry..."Come back, you cowards! Don't you guys like the smell of fear?"

From behind a monstrous oak tree, I peered out to see Dr. Rattacrackus casually stirring the flaming logs with the toe of his destroyed hip boots. Dr. Rat was not only pissed, but mentally deranged as well. After what seemed like an eternity, he turned from the fire and started walking, then trotting, from ground zero. What impeccable timing he had. As he started bee lining from the fire, the Gabers yelled in unison, "Run, Rat, Run!" sounding like a rodentian title to an Updike novel. As I pictured pieces of Rat all over the forest floor, I tried to imagine how I would explain Rat's demise to his mother, a highly excitable woman.

Sensing our urgency (and thus, his victory) and realizing the time for games was over, Rat started picking up the pace. As he streaked by us all, "KAABOOOM" the campfire exploded with a blinding white light. It had the force of a small thermonuclear explosion, engulfing the entire double deck gazebo and our summertime sleeping quarters in a giant fireball. With the sound of a hissing cobra, the steel propane cylinder chased Rat across the ground and between the trees like a cruise missile on auto kill. Moments later, there was only the darkness of the night, and the acrid smell of smoldering sleeping bags burning our nostrils. In the distant woods we heard the cry, not of Satan himself, but certainly one of his very best little helpers.

At The Lake we took other unbelievable risks with our lives and limbs. We were classic examples of youth's reckless "nothing can happen to me" attitude. You can imagine how we looked, climbing naked up a huge tree at the water's edge to dive into the shallows below. Tree diving, like everything else we did, was a challenge, a test of our abilities and courage. Each of us would climb higher than the one before until at last I found myself perched precariously in the top of the tree, inching my way over the water on a dangerously thin and wholly uncertain limb. When I was as high over the lake as I dared go, I felt my heart quicken in anticipation of the downward plunge. The branch bent under my weight as I approached its end and then threw me off as handily as the flick of a cow's tail scatters flies. I hit the water with a whoop and came up triumphant, after pulling my head up from the muddy bottom. I was sure this was how my life would be—filled with fun and adventure, danger and excitement—and sometimes mud. I was right.

One Saturday evening, patrons at the grand opening of the Millburn Diner became victims of a drive-by mooning at the hands, or should I say hams, of the "Men" led by Dr. Rattacrackus. I was in the lead car, the one that got away. The police caught them and dragged their big behinds in. The local judge, realizing that the success of the Millburn High School track team was now in his hands, declared that the butts in question were all of minor vintage. He tore up the citation that had been issued. Later, Rat wrote to me describing how his citation read. He wrote, "Wild Willy, I was given a moving violation for 'Hamming in a No Ham Zone'." Rat evoked a lot of emotions from the Gabers and me, but sympathy was not one of them.

WHAM!
Goss Boy Shot Stealing Old Volvo Bumper

"Don't move or I'll blow your head off!" A chill went coursing through my body and shocked my senses like an ice water injection.

Earlier that evening, on the way up to The Lake with Dan The Man ("The" being his middle name) and Gureenie, we passed a seedy-looking bar stuck back in the woods. Outside the bar was parked an old beat up 1965 Volvo 122S "Amazon," just like the one I had bought for $80. Only mine was an ugly piss-green color with the driver's side door smashed in. It's hard to believe Volvo would name a car model the Amazon, but they did. Each time we passed the bar, the car was there, always parked in the same place under the trees, looking to all the world as if it had been abandoned. One night I decided it was time to relieve that old Amazon of its back bumper. My car didn't have one, you see, and it was obvious to me, at least after a bottle of Boone's Farm Apple Wine, that whoever owned this one had no use for it.

My friends dropped me off near the bar and took off. The plan was for them to swing by to pick me up in a few minutes. As quietly as possible, I began to work at removing the prized bumper. I was well into my task when I felt the hair on the back of my neck stand up as I heard the deep voice, its tone agitated. My brain raced ahead, projecting the outcome of this encounter. I was going to die; or, if I didn't die I'd be caught stealing. That was worse, I decided, as my body broke out in a cold sweat that soaked my clothes. I could not embarrass my family by getting caught. I pictured *The New York Times* headline, "Goss Boy Shot Stealing Old Volvo Bumper." Another thought from the past blasted inside my head—I can't die this way—it's just too stupid!

I made my move. With one fluid motion I rose from my crouched position, bringing up my arm and knocking the shotgun out of the man's hands. In two bounds, I cleared a barbed wire fence and landed deep in the briar bushes and mud of a large, totally dark and unfamiliar swamp. I tore through the mud and underbrush and it tore through me. After what seemed like an eternity of crawling through the swamp, I neared the road. I thought I must be losing a pint of blood a minute to the mosquitoes that covered me, but I had no desire to make any noise by swatting them.

"Bless me Father for I have sinned." These words went through my head over and over again as I went to the famous last—but best—resort of people in serious trouble—prayer. "Lord, I know I'm a sinner, but you made me, so you already know that. Help me...PLEEAASE!!"

With that, I heard the familiar sound of Rat's beaten up, red Sunbeam Alpine convertible on its way back to pick me up. Rat always referred to it as "his spaceship from the planet Gwwaareeno." He sometimes put on the elaborate Martian costume of his infamous alter ego "Gordaan" and drove all over town providing free entertainment. I leaped out onto the highway and jumped into that beautiful old rust bucket. "Go! Go! Go!" I shouted to Dan The Man, who was driving.

"What da hell did you do?" Dan The Man asked. "You're covered with mud and bleeding all over da place."

The briars had destroyed me. My clothes were nearly torn off and my entire body was scratched and bleeding. I was covered from head to toe with mosquito bites. "That damn car belongs to some crazy mountain man with a shotgun," was all I could breathe out.

"Sure it does," Gureenie said, laughing.

"Yeah, ya butthole," Dan The Man added, "Ya chickened out, didn't ya? We knew you didn't have da nerve."

It took a few miles before I relaxed. After the terror of the moment had passed, Gureenie and Dan The Man started to believe my wild story. Gureenie said he would liked to have seen me clear the barbed wire fence, and if I could do that, why hadn't I been a track star. We decided Coach Boomer Beck should carry a shotgun as an incentive.

It was just after midnight when I turned around and saw the Volvo Amazon from the bar, pacing us about three car lengths back, running without its headlights on. "Holy shit, he's following us!"

Dan The Man's face turned white in the moonlight as he sped up. "Try to lose him, Dan," I said, my voice frantic. "Remember you're 'The Man'." During twenty minutes of Le Mans-like driving around hairpin turns cutting through the heavily wooded mountain pass, the animal driving the Amazon continuously pulled alongside us.

Still sans headlights, he rested a double barrel shotgun through his open passenger side window into the astonished face of Dan The Man and shouted for us to pull over "...before I blow your friggin' brains all over the place!!!" Dan followed the directions I shouted into his left ear and veered down a newly paved road. It worked! The Amazon missed our turn initially and blasted past us.

Instantly Gureenie screamed, "Not this way, Dan, no, no, no! Willy you big butthole!"

It was too late. The road quickly narrowed into a dead end forcing us to a terrifyingly sudden stop right in the middle of a remote, moonlit cornfield. It had been a wild ride—but now it was over.

"This is it," I thought as the speeding Amazon fishtailed directly in front of us across the narrow road and blocked our escape.

Shotgun first, the barechested, heavily muscled and profusely sweating man got out of his car. We were all too scared to run, although we wanted to. Anyway, he would have shot us in the back with no questions asked. He was that enraged, and he had every right to be.

Shaking violently, the man rested his gun's double barrel on the bridge of my nose. I stared down the two giant black holes like they were binoculars peering into my eternity. He exploded like an enraged demon, "Get out of the car!"

"Hey, he didn't mean anything, sir," Gureenie spoke out in my defense.

"Shut up!" the maniac screamed. His voice was out of control, his demeanor coldly determined. "Get out of the car!" I did as I was told, slowly and carefully climbing out of the back of the tiny red convertible.

"On your belly, boy!"

"No, sir," I said. Where did those words come from? Was I crazy, too? The man had a gun precariously perched on the bridge of my nose and he was absolutely out of his mind with anger. What were the odds I was going to survive this? No, he was going to kill me.

Again, he screamed. "Get down on your belly, boy!"

An ugly pig squealing scene from the movie *Deliverance* raced through my brain. "No, sir," I said again. The man was a hair trigger's twitch from blowing my face off. I had decided if I was going to die, it wouldn't be on my belly like one of my snakes. "You'll have to shoot me standing up if you're going to shoot me." I was determined not to let this guy have his way with me. The mosquitoes already had.

I'd like to tell you word for word what happened next, but I can't. I just started talking and talking and talking. An hour later I had talked my way right out of it. I wish I could remember today what I said that night. Gureenie and Dan The Man said I smoothed things over with that guy like homemade ice cream on a steaming hot day. For that they were grateful— eternally grateful. All I know is that the man didn't shoot me, and he could have. He didn't turn me in, and he should have. I swear I'm one lucky unlucky son of a gun, there's just no denying it.

CHAPTER TWO

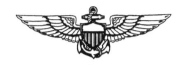

HIGHER EDUCATION COMES
IN MANY FORMS

Both my mother and my father were college graduates. It was a given that we would be, too, even though there were six kids in our good German-Irish Catholic family and significant amounts of money were hard to find—very hard. We all knew we'd have to finance our own way, but one thing we had all learned at an early age was the importance of a strong work ethic. I had been working for others since I was twelve years old to earn spending money. Still, college was another story, an expensive story, and it certainly seemed out of financial reach. Besides, school bored me and I needed a break from it. I had been having a great time and many of the Gabers wouldn't be college bound until the following fall.

Although I decided I wasn't going to go to college right away, it didn't take long to change my mind. I worked part-time as a garbage man, because the pay, the hours, and the exercise were all pretty good, at least from an eighteen-year-old's point of view. The veteran sanitation worker I assisted was handsome, healthy, and stunningly ignorant.

Once, when I dumped a can of garbage into the hopper of the truck, I saw his eyes get very wide. Then he reached deep into the hopper, something both very dangerous and very stupid to do, yet not out of character for him.

"Can't let this go to waste," he said, pulling out a greasy, smelly, half-eaten lobster tail from the nauseating heap. I watched in horror and disgust as he delightedly munched away while we hung precariously to the dump truck and it made its way up the street to the next stop. He explained as he ate that he wasn't stealing, this kind of perk was just one of the benefits that comes with the job—God Bless America—and so forth. This guy was a living testimonial to the infamous seafood diet—"I see food, I eat it." That moment changed my life. Then and there, I decided that I would go to college and I'd go right away. No need to delay.

I was accepted by the only school to which I applied, the University of Arizona. My brothers, Larry and Bobby, were students there. It may have been a case of the school not yet having reached its quota of idiots, (a maximum of one Goss boy per university ought to be a federal safety regulation, according to my friends). Mom was delighted. She wanted me to see that college academia wasn't so hard after all. She made me promise to go for at least a year before taking time off from the educational process. She didn't have to worry. This was the new Billy—post-lobster tail.

The first thing I did on arriving in Tucson was look for a job. I knew that if I didn't find one quickly, I'd head back home. After being there one week, I signed on as a weekend dynamiter in an underground copper mine about sixty miles distance from the university. For $4.13 an hour, I was allowed to swelter in stifling temperatures reaching upward to 120°F while creeping down narrow shafts a mile or so beneath the Earth's crust. It was an adventure, but a risky one, each time I entered the giant elevator that dropped at a rate of 2000 feet per minute into the 25 miles of underground tunnels. The humidity was so high you almost needed scuba gear, and the smell of burnt gunpowder could have choked a horse. The canaries had died long ago.

One hundred college students signed on with the mining company to work every Saturday and Sunday. After a few months only three of the original one hundred remained: Larry Rayko, David Pash and me. The others had long ago recovered their senses. Each evening, after coming up from a ball bustingly hard day's work, we were covered from head to toe with a heavy layer of brown muck. It took a long hot shower in the mine's massive locker room to get all that crud out of our hair, nose, eyes and skin. I'll never forget the toilets. There were about forty of them slammed into a giant white room with no cubicles or privacy screen. It provided little opportunity to take a relaxed crap which, I'm sure, was intentional. It seemed to be a blatantly designed disregard for human privacy and decency. Like everything else in my life, I would just have to grin and bear it.

My foreman in the mine thought I was a phenomenon of sorts because of my fairly large stature, light coloring and long blond hair. He may have been even a little suspicious of me. Typically, I'd be the only light-skinned Aryan idiot down there, surrounded by short, dark Mexicans who were dwarfed by my size. It wasn't a popular or comfortable social position for me but I got along okay. One thing in my favor was that the mine superintendent's last name was Goss. My co-workers thought we were related even though I had never met the man. His name saved me from being fired on more than one occasion.

Two of the Mexican workers used to call me the "Blond Chiquita" and were the funniest, grossest and most deviant little bastards I ever met, excluding Rat, of course. They would pinch my ass in the tight quarters of the double deck elevator. And, like some of the others, they would urinate through the corrugated steel mesh flooring onto the hard hats of the poor suckers below who hadn't been able to fight their way up to the top deck of the elevator. Believe me that was one place I tried to use my size and strength to my advantage. There was no way I would willingly let somebody pee on me. The mentality of some of the younger miners behind this particularly disgusting action seemed to be "What else is there to do for fun?" There didn't seem to be much else to do while riding the elevator in a mine shaft more than four times taller (or deeper) than the Empire State Building. You can imagine what it must have been like: a giant mass of filthy, stinking and dirty to the bone human flesh fighting through the line like steer in a cattle car to get a ride up on the top deck of that elevator. It was one helluva mess. After a hard day's work some of the veteran miners no longer even tried to fight their way to the top deck. They had been worn out, beaten, pissed and shit on their whole life. I guess to them it was no big deal.

Some of the hardest working, most dedicated and devoted God-fearing family men I have ever had the pleasure to know were miners with me. They had to be truly devoted to their families to do this job hour after hour, day after day, year after year. It was like toiling in hell—underground, hot as blazes, and humid as a swamp, swinging big sledgehammers and breaking huge rocks into smaller ones. It was really something to see, like a Herculean drama with the toils never ending—and as far removed from my previous life as a high school jock from the Jersey suburbs as could be imagined.

The routine was grueling, but paid enough for me to continue studying at the university. Monday through Friday, I would attend classes, study, socialize and generally have a good, and what I believed to be typical, college life. Then very early on Saturday and Sunday mornings I'd drive the 60 or so miles to the copper mine and drop down into the bowels of hell again. My training as a dynamiter consisted of only one morning's worth of instruction from an ex-professional wrestler who looked like his name, "Mr. Clean." He was an enormous bald man, immensely powerful, who could swing a huge twelve pound sledgehammer with one arm. Mr. Clean looked as if he had stepped right out of a freak show, especially when he drove the tiny electric mine train. He seemed more powerful than the motor itself, his giant legs straddling it like a little kid on a rocking horse. His instructions to me were always the same, "Goss, bust those boulders loose." Who was I to argue with him about the finer points of breaking rocks?

After a few months of closer than comfortable calls, I became pretty damn good with both a sledgehammer and the various kinds of explosives we used. The devices included stick dynamite, electronic blasting caps, bagged gunpowder and plastic explosives. There were rocks we wanted to break loose, and those we didn't. We lived in constant apprehension of an unplanned rock burst, where thousands of pounds of granite mixed with copper, gold and silver ore could break free and send us miners, collectively or individually, to a crashing, crushing, suffocating death. But sooner or later you got used to that fear as well.

During lunch break, the shift foreman liked to pull a bizarre stunt on us chuteblasters, as we were called. He'd take a head count to make sure no one had fallen asleep in one of the nearby chutes, then, when everybody was distracted with talk, or drinking hot coffee or soup, he'd hit the switch and instantaneously "KABOOOM!" A giant blast would rock the mine. We'd first hear the sound and then one to two seconds later we'd feel the compression as the activated switch simultaneously exploded all the electronically connected blasting caps in the thousands of pounds of dynamite, bagged gunpowder and plastic explosives we had laid out that morning. When the shock wave and air compression reached our lunch tunnel, only a moment after the explosion, the force of it would wring our diaphragms like a wet dishrag. The hollows of our body cavities were compressed so hard by the massive simultaneous explosion that whatever we had eaten, or had in our mouths, was violently expelled. If you happened to be facing someone at the time of the explosion—well, any friendship you may have developed pretty much ended right then and there. Your lunch partner's face would be covered with hot, half-digested food and drink. It was yours, and it wasn't pretty. Let me tell you, the walls in the eating tunnels were gross. Mine dining was definitely not fine dining.

I had a girlfriend back home. Alice was her name, and she was as nice a person as there could be. During breaks, I'd write her letters. Sitting on the rough, gravelly floor near one of the blasting chutes, I'd compose love letters and poems on equally rough toilet paper, using the bottom of my lunch box as a desk. She must have thought that was very romantic, don't you think? Her's was a generous and wealthy White Anglo-Saxon Protestant family that always treated me wonderfully. I'm not really sure her mother felt comfortable that her daughter received letters written on toilet paper from an earnest, longhaired Catholic boy who worked in an underground copper mine to put himself through school. Still, Mrs. Chrystie was always pleasant to me.

WHAM!
Goss Boy Found Dead in Town Dump

When Christmas break came around, I managed to get off from the mine long enough to make the trip to New Jersey to see Alice and my folks. It felt good to be home. It was a quiet and uneventful holiday until New Year's Eve, when the Gabers were gearing up for a big party at the Mueller's.

A few hours before I was to pick up Alice, my mother asked me to drive by the library parking lot and give my brother Bobby a lift home from his job in Millburn Center. The night was cold and dark, and the street lamps glowed with an eerie haze in the dampness of a misting rain. As I pulled behind the darkened library, I heard an unnatural sound, like a muffled scream, and slowed the car to a stop. Looking deeper into the darkness, I saw two elderly women. One was clinging desperately to her purse as she was viciously dragged across the pavement and knocked to the ground by a person twice her size. I drove up to the fallen woman and asked her companion if she was okay. As I jumped out of the car in pursuit of the attacker, I yelled back to the women, "I'll get that rotten son of a bitch!"

My brother Bobby had seen my car pull up as he approached

from across the street. He saw me jump out and run into the darkness. "I can't believe he'd hit you with the car and then run away," he told the woman, as he knelt to offer assistance.

"He didn't hit her, he's trying to catch the guy who did!" her bewildered friend responded. I had seen this guy's face only briefly, but recognized him as Tommy Green, a local doctor's son with a nasty reputation. He ran like hell and I ran after him in a full sprint that was hampered temporarily by the heavy winter clothes, which I shed while running into the freezing mist. My blood was boiling.

Tommy headed for the darkness, away from the brightly-lit parking lots and roadways. The chase went on at an exhausting sprint for well over a mile. He came to a trail by the railroad tracks and followed it. I followed him. The farther we went, the darker it became until all I could see was a flickering reflection of moonlight on the soles of his shoes and I could hear his footfalls echoing up ahead. Tommy had been a jock and was an all-around natural athlete who excelled at any sport he chose. Unfortunately, he had chosen losers for friends and drugs for recreation. He was a year younger than I was and in lean and powerful shape. I was fast, but I knew he was faster. I was strong, but he was also. I had no idea who would win the battle I was certain would follow if I caught him. But I was certain of one thing, whatever happened, it wasn't going to be pretty.

What worried me was that many drugs could give him both incredible strength and deadly resolve. I assumed he was on drugs that night, otherwise why would he do anything so brutal to an elderly lady? I knew that getting arrested on New Year's Eve was not one of Tommy's resolutions and he certainly would not surrender willingly. If I had been in his shoes I wouldn't have. These thoughts raced through my head as my pounding heart felt ready to explode as I tried to keep up with the speed demon. "The poor lady," I thought to myself, "he had been the predator and she the prey. Now I was the predator and he was the prey. What was he thinking? Did he know who was pursuing him?"

It looked to me like Tommy was headed for the town dump and he was probably thinking no one but a fool would follow him there. We were both right. That's where he headed, with one certified idiot in hot pursuit. What he didn't realize was that I knew the dump, its pitfalls and dangers, better than he did. I had worked for the Millburn Road Department as a garbage man.

When I finally worked my way through the bushes to the dump, the night was deathly still. I strained to hear Tommy moving or breathing among the shoulder-high evergreens that ringed the entrance. My own breath was tortured from the strain of the chase. Suddenly a shadowy figure stepped from behind a tree and quickly moved toward me. It was Tommy. My father's words echoed in my thoughts, "If you know someone's going to hit you—hit him first!" I lunged at Tommy, knocking him into the deep half-frozen mud, and I cut loose a primal scream which expressed my incredible rage over someone so privileged beating someone so defenseless.

Not expecting me to launch the first attack, an enraged Tommy and I fell to the ground breathing heavily and grappled on the rugged terrain of the dump. Ice and gravel cut into our frozen faces and hands as the Mother-of-All-Street-Fights began. Tommy threw me off his back with a solid elbow to my chin and kneed me in the ribs as he regained his feet. I grabbed his foot as he stood and twisted it, awkwardly stopping his escape and bringing him crashing down to the ground. His strength and resolve to flee at any cost had him continuously leaping to his feet, like a hooked tarpon, only to be yanked back down to the rugged surface again. After the long chase and an even longer struggle, we were both gasping furiously in the freezing air. Our muddied bodies were steaming and forming clouds in the winter cold like rutting bull elk with their antlers locked in deadly battle. This was for keeps and I was scared shitless. I knew I couldn't hold onto him much longer. What was he, or I, going to do next?

Patches of moonlight broke through the cloudy night, sending silvery ghost-like glimpses of the mugger to my eye. Blow for blow, we swung at each other for what seemed an eternity, tasting each other's spit, blood and hair. At first I fought for the elderly woman. Then, I fought for justice for all humanity. At the end, I fought for my own life.

Then, I realized I was running out of strength and time. This maniac was now trying to kill me and if I didn't end this soon, he would succeed. It wasn't enough anymore for him to simply escape. He knew me. He knew I knew him. He came from a well-to-do and respected family. He was a doctor's son. He could not take the chance of recognition or arrest. He would kill me with his bare fists if necessary or any weapon he could find. It might take days for anyone to find my body. With waning energy, I realized that he was again the predator and I the prey. The realization gave me added resolve and I wrestled him to the ground once more. We had learned from some of the same wrestling coaches and knew the same moves, but I managed to get on top and hold him, at least for a moment.

As Tommy groped along the ground with his free hand, he found a heavy stick with a ragged, pointed end. I barely saw it coming in the pale moonlight as he blasted it straight upward, with the hopes of impaling my forehead or eye. Pure luck and instinct made me turn my head a fraction to the right as it grazed the side of my left ear, almost taking out my eye. It stunned me to realize he had deliberately tried to blind me. Until that moment, I had been trying to immobilize him rather than hurt him. Now, with the near loss of an eye, my focus shifted. His desperate attempt to blind me was the final blow, the proverbial straw that broke the camel's back. No more Mr. Nice Guy.

I was now empowered with an unnatural energy reserve that gave me the strength to lift him off the ground and run him head first into the massive fieldstone wall that edged one side of the dump. Three times I rammed his head into that wall, but I could not knock him unconscious. I felt my endurance fail, and began to pray silently for enough strength not to pass out. I prayed for Tommy to give up while we were both still alive. I was terrified.

Finally, collapsed together by the wall, I heard the words that I had been praying for. "Yu-you win—I gi-give up," Tommy said, exhausted and beaten.

"Oh my God! Now what?" I thought, knowing no one would be looking for us behind the locked gates and wooded periphery of the town dump. I didn't for a second trust Tommy to stay put, and I didn't have anything to tie him up with or to prevent his escape. It seemed to take forever as I half dragged half pushed him through the darkness, mud and bushes onto Main Street. It didn't take long to realize I was right not to trust him. Although Tommy had verbally given up, he was still struggling to get away. The guy had always had a reputation for being very strong but in my weakened state he seemed superhuman.

There was little traffic on the brightly-lit road. I knew I could go no farther, so I pushed Tommy's face up against a splintery telephone pole and forced him to sit on the ground with his legs straddling the pole. Then I sat down close behind him with my legs tightly wrapped around his back and the telephone pole. After doing that, I wrapped his arms around the pole and clutched his opposing wrists, turning myself into a human straight jacket sandwiching him between the telephone pole and my body. In that unlikely position, covered in freezing blood, sweat, and piss, I waited for the police to hurry up and arrive before I passed out.

I was hoping they'd show up immediately, but instead, a woman walking her dog first appeared. Tommy spotted her, too. "Hey, Lady!" he called out, "Get this guy off me, he's crazy. Sic your dog on him!"

"Call the police!" I countered. "He's lying! He just mugged a woman!"

The woman ran away, looking very confused, but a few minutes later two police cars pulled up. The officers got out of their squad cars and stared in amazement at two ruggedly built teenage boys locked together like mating toads against a telephone pole. They had never before seen this technique of immobilizing a suspect. We were so cold; they nearly needed a crowbar to separate us. Unsure as to which one of the two longhaired youths to arrest they sped off to the station with both of us.

Tommy claimed I attacked him. I stated I had seen him attack an elderly woman. The woman, I learned later, was from France, and her companion was too dazed and confused to assist the police with the identification of the assaulter. I guess all longhaired American white boys look the same to a French lady. Fortunately, after a little time, she recognized my voice and my story was declared to be true. The doctor's son was arrested, found guilty of atrocious assault and battery, with attempted robbery thrown in, and I was given a police citation on a nice wooden plaque for bravery. Also, the mayor sent me a letter, which made my parents proud.

Oh, and in spite of all the trouble, the fight, the police reports and the injuries, Alice and I made it to that New Year's Eve party. And it was a blast.

One of my roommates while in college was Doug "Snakeman" Finnegan. Snakeman arrived at Apache Hall with a bulging, wriggling pillowcase. Instantly, I recognized it as a pillowcase full of snakes, so I knew I was going to get along great with this guy no matter what. Once a month, whether we needed it or not, we'd go on a snake hunt in the nearby Sonoran Desert, taking along Harvey Perkins, our buddy across the hall.

Snakeman and I got along famously, and spent a week together at his wealthy grandfather's getaway house on a mountaintop in San Mateo, California, overlooking San Francisco Bay. When we first drove the old Volvo Amazon up to the gate of the rarely visited estate, Snakeman, Harvey Perkins and I were met by several large, dark-suited men in sunglasses.

"FBI," they said, flashing their badges in our faces.

"What the hell did I do now?" I wondered. The charming and highly efficient California State Police had just ticketed me twice in the past hour on the way there. The nation's highways had just unilaterally adopted a too-slow 55-mph speed limit and I was convinced the liberal state of California was ticketing every out-of-state licensed car driven by a longhaired person.

Anyway, it now appeared that one-way discussions with official looking men were unfortunately starting to become the norm for me on this trip. With the operative words "Yes, sir" strategically placed throughout a conversation that sounded something like this:

"You three longhairs stay put tonight—understand?"

"Yes, sir!"

"We mean it, don't go anywhere—understand?"

"Yes, sir. What happened, sir?"

"None of your damn business, son—understand?"

"Yes, sir!"

While most people use the word "understand" as a means to ask as a question, my buddies and I discovered that the FBI had an entirely different way of using the word—as an order.

Once safely inside the beautiful hilltop retreat, we heard on the radio that a young heiress had been kidnapped from her home just down the street from where we were staying. Were Snakeman, Harvey and I suspects, even for a moment, in the kidnapping of Patty Hearst? Probably so.

WHAM!
Goss Blown Up in Mine Explosion

As an adult, I continued facing near-death experiences. Was I lucky, unlucky, stupid, brave or a tenacious combination?

A friend of mine, Mollie Marchev, asked me to take her roommate to a campus sorority party. Blind dates were not something I was prone to accept, but being an eternal optimist, I figured it would be all right this time since Mollie was pretty good looking and I thought good looking girls kind of hung around together. Boy, was I wrong! Her towering roommate thundered down the stairs and almost crushed my hand on introduction. "Bill, how da hell ya doin'?" she said as she threw her meat cleaver arm around me, drawing me close to her like a female praying mantis preparing her mate for his first—and last—fling.

Thinking ahead, she had brought along a shopping bag full of tequila to loosen me up. Normally, I liked to stay sober on first dates, but there was nothing normal about this date. That night I obliged her by drinking all of it. The party got pretty wild, and I was in heaven, though not with my date. The objects of my attentions and affections were her sorority sisters. I didn't get home until four in the morning. I had a great time!

When Larry Rayko picked me up for the drive to the mine a few hours later, I didn't have a hangover. I was still drunk. I was also late, which, to a mining operation, is an unforgivable condition (unlike being drunk or hungover). Being late held up the carefully timed elevator drops, yet you could work with a hangover. Apprehensively, I approached the foreman.

"You're fired, Goss."

"Please let me work. I'm sorry I'm late. Please give me another chance. I promise it won't happen again."

He looked at me with an unforgiving eye. "Please," I begged. "I need this job."

I thought for a moment then appealed to his macho side, "I was in a sorority house full of beautiful women last night, and I lost track of time. Boss, I know how you appreciate the ladies. I'm sure you understand."

Without a word he nodded reluctantly and waved me off in the direction of the elevator shaft. Almost being fired had sobered me up and a dull headache began to flirt behind my eyes. It teased its way across my forehead, then settled on top of my head like a carpenter's vise. There was no relief and there was none in sight. It hurt and I realized this would be the longest ten-hour day I might ever experience.

At the five thousand-foot underground level I came to a

plugged chute off to the side of a forty-foot deep hole. The clog was an unusually large rock cluster weighing thousands of pounds that blocked the chute a dangerous twelve feet up from the opening. I readied the dynamite and blasting caps, then, as an afterthought, I hooked my safety line to the cable overhead, something miners do only rarely because it slows things down too much to disconnect and reconnect it every twenty feet. This time, I did it to appease my Spanish-speaking foreman, who was giving me a spot safety check. My breath came in short, hot gasps in the dank, acrid air of the mine. The pressure in my head was building and the familiar pounding of a world class hangover was beginning in my ears. I maneuvered bags of gunpowder and sticks of dynamite on a ten-foot long wooden pole, poking it among the unstable boulders over my head.

I had just completed wiring the blasting caps and was about to step back and admire my work when I heard the dreaded "crack" of shattering granite, sounding like the supersonic crack of a rifle bullet. It was followed immediately by the muffled crashing noises of a rock burst directly above and behind me. There was barely time to turn as thousands of pounds of unstoppable granite boulders, the ones I was working to dislodge, crashed into the bags of blasting powder, sticks of dynamite, blasting caps—and me. I was hit on the left knee, swept off my feet and knocked silly. As I began to recover my senses, I heard the sound of giant steel trap doors below me, jarring large rocks like ping pong balls in a bingo machine and dropping them into the mine's train cars on the level below us. I was suspended in mid-air, hanging by a nylon umbilical cord over the mouth of the gaping forty-foot hole. I had been saved from the giant steel jaws of the deadly trap doors by the horizontally run safety wire I had just hooked onto during the spot safety check. From the looks of it, I hadn't needed to set up any dynamite at all: I could have yelled at those damn rocks and the vibration of my voice would have brought them down. Chute blasting was part science, part art. And although I had followed the science part to a tee, the art part had just about killed me.

I regained full awareness before my foreman sat me up against the wall of the dark, damp tunnel. "I thought you were a goner, mon," said my Mexican foreman. "Dat big rock knocked you up and out of da way—you shoulda been sandwiched like a damn granite taco, mon. You one lucky blond Chiquita, mon." My head was pounding and my body ached. All I wanted was to get the hell out. I tried to get up. "Just lie still, mon, be quiet a minute. You be hurt maybe. I be back in a little while." He was a good mon....

I closed my eyes, thanking God the dynamite hadn't blown the moment it got smashed under the rockslide and I wondered if any parts of me were broken or missing. Then I decided it didn't matter, I was getting out of this hellhole for good. This was too tough a way to make a living and there was no future in it—I'd probably die before getting a fifty-cent raise. With more than a little effort, I stood, turned my headlamp off and studied the unbelievable blackness of the mine one last time. As my eyes acclimated to the lack of light, I saw the tiny shadow of a man swinging his giant sledgehammer. It danced on the wall behind him like some distant devil and gave me a lasting impression forever etched into my brain. Later, as the sunlight kissed my face when the elevator busted through to the surface of the earth, I felt as if I'd been touched by the Lord himself. I limped stiffly over to the shift foreman's shack after I showered up and stuck my head inside. "I quit."

"What do you mean you quit?" he shouted after me as I hobbled to my car. "Aren't you the guy who begged me to let you keep your job? Wasn't that just this morning?" I kept walking.

WHAM!
Goss Feared Lost on Mt. Lemon

Having escaped death in the depths of the earth, the next weekend I had a close call when hiking in the mountains. You could say I went from one extreme to the other. Several of my college friends and I decided to hike the snowy-peaked 10,000-foot Mt.

Lemon outside Tucson, Arizona. Our intentions were good. We'd drive to the top, leisurely hike the fifteen miles or so down to Sabino Canyon, camp overnight, fish and swim in a spectacular mountain spring and generally enjoy the great outdoors. There were nine of us, four guys, four girls and a dog named Hazel. Personally, my left knee was still a bit sore from my experience in the mine the week before. As a group, we were completely unprepared for what was to happen.

None of us had a flashlight. None of us carried more than a small canteen of water. None of us had hiking shoes. None of us even wore long pants! Sunscreen was not an issue. The only item in good supply was tequila, and we had plenty of that. We were happy college kids on an adventure, dressed in our shorts and sandals and ready for a dream come true.

When we saw the snow cresting the top of this behemoth in the desert, we were exhilarated. Spirits were high as we started our trek from the top walking on the thin wispy snow in the warm glorious light of the noonday sun.

The guy who took the car back down the mountain to meet us the next day was jealous that he'd drawn the short straw. Actually, he turned out to be the lucky one. Within hours of our venture deeper into the woods, the trail became less prominent. It was poorly marked, and soon we were not-such-happy college kids totally lost as the cool shadows of the towering pines merged into the rapidly changing hot and cold of the desert mountain terrain. We were clueless as to what happened to the trail.

The first night, we kept each other's hopes alive with stories of how easy it would be to find the trail again when the sun came up, how cooperative the weather was and how really beautiful it was on the mountain. It was cold and we stayed close to each other, sleeping fitfully in spite of our cheerful words.

Sometime during the night, BB, the leader of this ship of fools, fractured his kneecap trying to break a piece of ironwood in half for the fire. I had been amazed to see him get ready to attempt another crack over his knee after being so thoroughly unsuccessful at that first crack, but the tequila was making him brave. The second try at breaking the wood did him in and I thought it somewhat comforting to find a nineteen-year-old ego even bigger than mine. Impressing women should always fall short of hurting yourself, but do give it your best shot. In that, BB could be proud. The next day we found a dry streambed and began to follow it, feeling certain it would lead us down the mountain to Sabino Canyon. Cactus and nettles tore at our legs and clothing as we made our way through the deep ravines. Gigantic twenty-foot high boulders often blocked our path along the river gulch. We'd hardly eaten for almost thirty hours, and found only tiny pockets of dirty water along the way. My longtime friends Derry and Debby's faces reflected the fear and stress we all felt.

BB's knee was giving him hell and although we were able to splint it and somewhat relieve his pain, it was sobering to all of us. We began to realize how very vulnerable we were, and an unspoken fear joined our group. The trek became torturously slow, confronted with one enormous boulder after another. Often we were unable to cover more than a mile in three hours. Hazel's foot pads were wearing off and bleeding from the brutal terrain, and I finally had to sling her around my neck and carry her. Hungry and tired, we all cheered when we finally saw in the distance a large clearing, which from afar looked like Sabino Canyon. On reaching its edge, however, we suddenly discovered that the clearing was, in actuality, a cliff that dropped 400 feet to a clear flowing stream below, our first clean-looking water. I knew the stream would eventually lead us downhill to our destination and we desperately needed that water, if only we could climb down the cliff. Plus, BB had already inadvertently dropped his knapsack to the bottom of the cliff, where it lay exploded like a smashed June bug.

"I'll try it," I said to the others, "and let you know if it's safe."

"Don't do it, Bill, it looks too dangerous," said Derry.

"Well, we can't stay up here," Amy commented. "Maybe we should all go down together."

"BB can't do that with his knee," Brownie replied. "Someone will have to stay here with him, and we'll send back for you. How about you, Debby?"

"You should all stay right here until I check it out," I answered. "There's no reason for all of us to risk our necks."

"Listen to the miner. He knows about rocks."

"Hey, let him go, I certainly don't want to be the guinea pig."

I lowered myself off the side of the cliff and groped with my feet for a rock ledge I had seen from above. Finding it, and feeling it secure, I eased one hand down and to the side, seeking something to hold. Step by tortured step, I crawled down the cliff side, imagining I must look like the vampire Dracula creeping down his castle walls.

Halfway down, I was tempted to yell up to the others to join me when the rock that was supporting my weight suddenly popped loose from the face of the cliff. "Oh shit!" I thought as I momentarily balanced on my left toe, holding onto nothing but a useless rock, looking down at a 200-foot drop to the creek bed below.

"This is it," was all I could muster as I tossed the worthless rock over my left shoulder and started my backward treefall. A friend's brother had died exactly this way a few years earlier— I guess I hadn't learned anything from it. Desperately, I reached forward for something, anything that would return me to my previous bat-like position pressed snugly against the cliff. Out of the corner of my eye I spotted a peanut-sized snake hole directly beneath the rock that had popped free. At the speed of light my left index finger found it—PAY DIRT! I dug my finger deep into the hole like a kid after a sand crab at the beach, holding on by my one finger, literally, for dear life. I heard Derry scream and knew she was looking down at me. I closed my eyes and prayed that my aching finger would hold and that some snake wouldn't try to dislodge it from his den or try and eat it or have its way with me. What a time to think about sex.

After my heart stopped racing, I once again resumed my descent. The sun was fading and it was getting harder to find the hidden steps that would free me from being trapped on the cliff's face in total darkness. Going too fast would kill me but going too slow would be just as dangerous as the sun was setting behind the mountain peak. I didn't have a lot of options. I couldn't climb up again because the rock that popped free was an essential foothold to the top. By the time I reached the streambed below, it was completely dark. When the sun sets in a mountain canyon, it becomes pitch black almost immediately. I could hear Derry crying, but couldn't see her. She had somehow become separated from the others when the sun fell below the mountaintop creating instant nighttime. Poor Derry was trapped in the darkness alone on a desert ledge.

"It's okay, Derry, it's going to be okay," I called up. "But you can't come down this way, it's way too dangerous."

It was so dark that to take another step risked breaking an ankle or leg, or worse, falling to an untimely death. So I yelled up to my friends they'd have to settle in where they were till the morning light. I dwelled on how we'd get the body out if someone fell. I listened to Derry crying all night long, her sobs chopping into my soul like tiny hatchets. I began to fear her tears would destroy her, and maybe me, too. From time to time, she'd cry out in fright terrified of the animal eyes that encircled her on her cliff side perch. They probably belonged to coatimundi, large raccoon-like creatures that traveled the desert in packs. These animals were not necessarily vicious, but not necessarily friendly either.

I knew what Derry felt, for I had felt it. She was convinced she was going to die right there on the side of Mt. Lemon. It was supposed to be a fun time, a leisurely trip, and now she was going to die. She was one of the gutsiest and smartest girls I knew, but this was just too stupid. It made her cry out loud. If Derry fell asleep, she could end up dead. We both knew that.

And I would do everything within my power to help her stay awake. And she did.

"The coatis probably won't eat you, Derry," I called up to her, encouraging her, scaring her, whatever it took to keep her awake through the night and discourage her from trying to climb out in the darkness. She was not amused. I told her jokes and sang songs and called out to her throughout the black night until the morning light made the "eyes" go away and she could relax. What a trooper!

After sunrise, Derry and the others were able to find their way down a less steep part of the mountain and all nine of us, including Hazel the dog, reunited. They were all covered with hundreds of cactus spines, as their climb back up to the top of the mountain ridge had proved almost as dangerous as my climb down. That evening we finally stumbled upon our destination, the ever-popular Sabino Canyon. We looked for all the world like shipwreck survivors. Having lost most of our gear on the cliff, including our sleeping bags, we just crawled on by the bikini-clad vacationers, desperate to get back to our dorms, desperate for a hot shower.

Derry heard her phone ringing as she unlocked the door to her dorm. "What's the matter... are you okay?" her mother hysterically asked her. The night before Derry's father awoke with a frightened start, at the exact same moment that Derry had started crying alone on her cliffside perch. Her mom and dad, 2500 miles away, instantly knew their daughter was in trouble. Coincidence? Maybe, but unlikely. The Russian government has been investigating ESP for decades in the hopes of discovering a new secret weapon. Perhaps all they need to do is talk to a few parents whose kids are away from home on weekend camping trips.

After both surviving and completing my freshman year at the University of Arizona, in my case quite an unexpected accomplishment, I returned to New Jersey and resumed my long-standing friendships with my fellow Gabers. Our experiences were always adventurous and memorable, especially when Rat was involved.

That fall, Rat and I drove the Volvo Amazon up to New Hampshire to attend a Halloween party that Jim "Jungle James" Mardis was having. During our visit, Jim took Rat and me to a giant mountain gorge and pointed up several hundred feet to a condemned railroad trestle that stretched across it. Class IV and V whitewater rapids ran headlong through the gorge below.

We climbed up the mountainside to the edge of the dilapidated railroad trestle. Jim looked at us. "Hey, follow me gents, I want to show you something."

I responded, "Come on Jim, what are you nuts? We can't cross that thing—it's falling apart."

All Jim said was "Yup" and he started inching along the trestle to get to the other side. Rat gave me his standard look that says, "We've done stupider things, I just can't remember when." Off he went with me following close behind. If there was ever a time not to have a fear of heights, this was it. The trestle creaked and buckled but never gave way and some girls took pictures as we crawled across it like slugs, only slugs are smarter.

When we got to the end, I said, "Jim what the hell did you want to show us?"

"Just this, Wild Willy, the other side," he responded. Rat and I refused to recross the trestle to get back to our car so the Jungle in Jim came out again, "Well, boys we'll just have to swim it then."

"Jimmy," Rat said, "There is no way in hell we can swim those rapids without getting swept down that waterfall below."

"Sure there is," he said. "Follow me." He led us down the side of the gulch to the river's edge. "There's an underwater cable that we can hold onto as we cross."

"Come on Jimmy—that's crazier than the trestle crossing!" I said, totally flabbergasted.

"I love it," Rat responded. So like three idiots with our testicles wrapped around our Adam's apples, we plunged into the frigid water of that wide whitewater river. Somehow we pulled ourselves across to the other side using a cable that looked electrical in nature. Believe me, the word's out on Jungle James. When he says, "Follow me," there usually aren't any takers.

That night, after the costume party, Doctor Rat and I drove the Amazon, which I had affectionately named "Festus," to visit my sister Peggy at a sorority party. It was an unusually warm October and as we drove the old 65 Volvo along the dark waterfront of Lake Winnipesaukee, we saw all sorts of bumps in the road. Big ones, small ones, moving ones—wait a minute—moving ones? It turned out to be a massive nighttime frog and toad migration.

Rat got that faraway look in his eyes and I knew immediately what he was thinking. I pulled Festus over and we started loading up as many frogs and toads as possible. We had at least one hundred of the little cold-blooded critters in various sizes and shapes, approximately the rated amphibian load for a two-door Volvo Amazon. Rat held the Mother of all Bullfrogs on his lap for "that special occasion." I looked at Rat's beady little eyes, "No, probably not Satan himself, but certainly one of his most special little helpers," I again thought to myself and smiled. Whatever he had in mind, one thing was sure, this was going to be fun.

The sound in the car was thunderous from the bullfrogs' jugarums, the toads' croaks and the peepers' peeps. The smell of frog sweat, which I'm certain they don't have, was unusually strong. If I were going to come down with a bad case of warts, this would be the night.

We got to the sorority and it was a packed house, packed with drunken women that is. I met my sister Peggy and she could tell we were up to no good. "Billy, I don't want to know what you have planned, just give me plenty of time to get out of here before you do it."

"Better start running now, Sister," I said.

Rat and I found some pizza boxes and filled each with about twenty amphibians. We then carried the boxes inside the sorority house going from room to room putting live toads in cosmetic kits, cookie jars, medicine cabinets, closets, book bags, and under telephone handsets. "Every amphibian has its place," Rat mused, mimicking a former grammar teacher discussing dangling participles.

As we headed downstairs, we noted the massive line to the downstairs lavatory—all girls of course—since any self-respecting college guy would be peeing outside in the woods.

"Wild Willy," Rat gleefully exclaimed, it's now time for the secret weapon—AMPHIBOMB!" He went out and came in again, holding a giant lump under his sweatshirt. He then faked severe nausea, a performance which was so good that it immediately earned him head of the line privileges to the john. In he went and out he came, sans bump under sweater, tearfully holding back laughter as he thanked the gorgeous, buxom blonde who kindly had let him butt in line. As she went in, Doctor Rat whispered in my ear a very visual presentation of what was going on behind that closed bathroom door.

"Willy, bathroom light switch comes on, but no light turns on, because I loosened the light bulb. Toilet seat cover comes up in darkness, shorts come down to ankles, butt presses firmly in place on toilet seat. Now...listen carefully...there it is...the sound of warm tinkle on the head of a cold bullfrog—AMPHIBOMB!"

At that precise moment, a bloodcurdling shriek echoed throughout central New Hampshire as Rat led the way out the front door in an almost catatonic state of mischief nirvana. The following morning my sister Peggy asked us if we knew anything about it. Rat and I stuck our hands in our pockets and looked at the ground, unwilling to confess to the frogging of Kappa Kappa Gamma.

WHAM!
Goss Breaks Neck on Concrete Floor

The summer after my first year of college, I spent time with Jeff Marcketta, or Boobus, as everyone called him. Boobus and I were big buddies. At 300 pounds, Boobus was a bigger buddy to me than I was to him. One night, we decided to go pay a visit to Sandy "Stench a la Foof" North, at Fairleigh Dickinson (a.k.a. "Fairly Ridiculous") University. Foof was a fantastic wrestler made even more famous by his ability to fake injuries thus allowing himself time to catch his breath. His naive opponents, genuinely believing he had a real injury, would try to capitalize on it, leaving themselves open to defeat, which inevitably happened.

As Boobus and I prepared that night to make a Stench run to Fairly Ridiculous, my father sensed trouble. "Listen, Billy," he said, "You're going into the Navy soon so don't do anything stupid tonight. Just try and show up back home in one piece, will you, son?"

I gave him the standard father/son reply, "Yeah, sure, Dad," and off Boobus and I went. Undoubtedly, we had that Friday night gleam in our eyes, the same gleam that strikes terror in the souls of fathers with teenage boys everywhere.

Two hours later I was wrestling Stench on the concrete floor of his dormitory. I was doing fine considering how much slower the vodka had made my reflexes. As I was getting ready to slide in for another double leg takedown, I suddenly went airborne straight to the ceiling. Boobus, gigantic, immensely strong and highly intoxicated—held my life—my fragile, stupid little life—in his hands which were stretched over his head about eight feet above the concrete floor. I spread my arms like a bird, feeling safe and comfortable in the grasp of this friendly behemoth, but the vodka had altered his judgment as well. Proving his strength, he tossed me like a fly without wings. It was the start of a long history of me logging flight time. Not expecting to be suddenly airborne while in the hands of such a close friend my pearly whites hit the concrete floor with the full force of 185 pounds behind them. CRACK!

What was remarkable to all the pre-med students in the room was that only my front teeth were shattered and not my entire spinal column. I also had a deep split in the skin from my left nostril to my mouth that caused a steady stream of mucus to run from my nose into my mouth. Needless to say, it wasn't pretty.

I'll never forget my phone call to Dad that night, nor do I doubt will he. "Dadf, I fink I scwooed up," I muttered through my busted teeth.

"Yeah, I think you did," muttered my Dad, secretly delighted that it was only a visit to the dentist and not the police station or the morgue.

Boobus more than made up for my broken teeth. That year, he and his girlfriend Bonnie introduced me to Peggy Gleason. Bonnie and Peggy worked together as waitresses, first at an ice cream shop and later at an Italian restaurant named Marco Polo, while they both put themselves through college.

Peggy had a perfect face and the most incredible little body I'd ever seen. "Lord, what a bonus it would be if she's nice, too," I thought. Once again, my prayers were answered. There goes that luck again.

One of the first times I saw Bill—I don't call him Billy—in action was at a movie theater. I was with my friend Bonnie, who was going with Jeff Marcketta, and the two of them had been trying to fix me up with this guy, Billy Goss, for a couple of weeks.

"You'll love him, Peggy," Bonnie said, "He's such fun to be with, so outrageous!"

"And why do you think I'd want to be with somebody outrageous?" I countered.

"I think you need that. You've been such a mess lately since you broke up with Chip. Acting so depressed all the time. You don't ever have any fun anymore. You need a guy like this, Peg, why not

give it a try? Just agree to meet us with him one time, that's all. He doesn't even have to know it's been arranged."

So I agreed, and found myself at the movies. Bill and Jeff were already seated when Bonnie and I came in. The movie hadn't started and the theater lights were still shining brightly, or at least they seemed bright when I saw my date. He was casually sitting back in his seat with his western-booted feet firmly up on the back of the seat in front of him, and he was cloaked in an easy-going, "devil may care" air of total confidence. I was horrified.

The thoughts that ran through my mind threw me into an emotional turmoil. First of all, I was embarrassed that he was sprawled out in the theater seat with his feet up like that. It was such a rude thing to do and certainly not how I was raised. Next, I was angry that I had let Jeff and Bonnie convince me to meet this guy. But when he said hello, and his smile was so warm, I thought I'd melt. I decided to stay.

Bill talked and laughed, and not quietly either, all the way through the movie which was the incredibly goofy Blazing Saddles. *I shrank down in my seat and hoped no one would see me. After the movie, I really wanted to escape, but he kept talking—about himself. "What an ego," I thought. When I saw Bonnie the next day, I wanted to choke her.*

"Well?" she asked me excitedly.

"Well, what?"

"Well, what did you think of Billy?"

"What do you think I thought?" I answered, letting my irritation show. "He's overly loud and incredibly obnoxious. Definitely not my type. I can't believe I let you talk me into going out with him."

"Well, he likes you."

"How can you tell? All he ever talks about is himself."

"He just does. He'll call. You'll see."

"I'll try not to be home," I said laconically.

"Come on, Peggy," Bonnie said, "He's a good looking guy with an adventurous nature. It won't hurt you to loosen up a little. When he calls, give him a chance, maybe some of his positive attitude will

rub off on you."

I didn't answer, but I did think about what she'd said. It was true I had been less than enthusiastic about most things, and really a little pessimistic about most everything. When Bill asked me out again, I accepted. He was always very nice, and totally upbeat. We went out a few times over the summer, although I don't know why he kept asking me out since I wasn't very warm to him most of the time.

I knew he also dated other girls, one fairly regularly, but he never talked about her. I was glad he had a girlfriend, actually, since I could only take him in small doses and I had absolutely no intention of ever letting things become serious between us. A little bit of Bill Goss went a long way with me and I knew he was not the man of my dreams. An interesting diversion, maybe, but nothing long term.

All the time we dated that summer, Bill never pressured me for anything. He was always a very physical person and I know he must have wanted to get things going a lot faster with me than we did. I guess you could say he was a gentleman in that respect. I was pretty impressed when he remembered my birthday, and I really admired the way he never let any kind of obstacles get in his way. He was a very "can-do" type guy, and I began to think of him as a confidant. He made me laugh, and cry, and look at life differently. We became friends.

"Love doesn't make the world go 'round.
Love is what makes the ride worthwhile."
— Franklin P. Jones

"Don't concentrate on trying
to prove your abilities.
Instead, concentrate on trying
to improve your abilities."
—E. J. Goss

Chapter Three

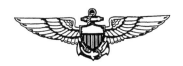

IN THE NAVY: ROUND ONE— MINEMAN GOSS

"I *'ve decided what I'm going to do next, Peg," Bill said. We were across the counter from each other at a local ice cream shop where I worked. He was eating an ice cream sundae, for free, of course.*

"Going back to school?" I asked, assuming the answer would be yes. He had spent a year at the University of Arizona and it was natural to think he'd continue, even though he hadn't taken any steps in that direction over the summer and had been working as a welder at TiFab, a titanium plant in northern New Jersey.

Bill shook his long golden hair. "Nope, I'm going to join the Navy." My face must have gone white, because he looked at me with sudden alarm. "Are you okay?"

I recovered. "I should be asking you that," I answered. "Are you crazy? You don't have the personality to be controlled like that, to have people telling you what to do and when and how. It's just not you, Bill—what about your mother? You know she wants you to finish college."

"Oh, I'll finish, but next time I'll let the G.I. Bill pay for it." He paused. "I want the adventure, the travel. I want to see the world. My mother won't mind. Being a travel agent, she's always encouraged the wanderlust in all of us. It's an opportunity to do something for myself and to make a contribution to the country. I'm willing to trade a little control for a lot of adventure."

We sat in silence for a moment while I absorbed what he had said. I was shocked at first because the military was not normally looked upon as an option in our part of the country. In northeastern New Jersey, kids out of school didn't enlist in the Navy or anything else unless they were forced to. The armed services just wasn't a part of our lives. There were no military bases nearby, there was no military population. We rarely saw people in military uniforms and we certainly didn't understand anything about it. Young men out of high school or college got a job; they were bankers, doctors or salesmen. Most people thought if you enlisted in the service, you must have done something wrong. If that was Bill's case, I sure didn't know what it was. But once I thought about it, joining the Navy was probably a pretty smart thing for Bill to do. He could have his adventure and plenty of travel, see places he might never get to see otherwise, and then come home to an assured education.

Most of our friends reacted the same way I did. They thought he was crazy at first, then warmed to the idea. I never knew what Bill's other girlfriend thought of it, yet I felt they were drifting apart. He didn't speak of her often; of course, that may have simply been his considerate nature. I knew she had been traveling a lot overseas with her family. That may even have been an influence in Bill's decision to join the Navy and see the world. It seemed that many of his friends and family members were going to exciting places outside the country and he wasn't. And Bill wasn't the kind to let the fact that he didn't have much money curb his appetite for travel or anything else for that matter.

Bill left for Basic Training in Orlando, Florida, right before Christmas. His chosen specialty? Underwater explosives—he was going to be a mineman. It seemed a little ironic, Bill going from one kind of mine to another—from the depths of the earth to the depths of the sea. The day he left, his father almost cried, which was very telling to me. His dad was a man who was never at a loss for words, who exuded confidence with a tough but fun-loving nature that made you glad to be around him. He was a Coast Guard veteran of World War II and his four years on the high seas of the Pacific and Caribbean were some of his most memorable. Yet, on this particular day he could hardly express himself. I could tell he *was very, very proud of his son.*

Bill and I began to write to each other and our friendship grew. We really got to know each other through those letters. I was the pessimist and he was the optimist. It was spooky how he always seemed to know just what to say. Many times as I would read and re-read his letters, I'd think he was inside my head, thinking my thoughts and putting them in order for me. It was amazing how close I began to feel to this incredibly obnoxious, overly loud, totally upbeat, paradoxically sensitive and caring egomaniac. Still, I was a long, long way from being romantically involved with him. He just wasn't my type. It was remarkable that our system of values was the same—remarkable.

From Orlando, the Navy sent Bill to Charleston, South Carolina, to train as a mineman, and then to Long Beach, California. I'd meet the mailman, hoping for another bizarre episode in the life of Bill Goss. His letters always had a lot of substance and humor. They were fun to read.

I enlisted in the Navy while the Vietnam War dragged on, thanks in part to a spineless Secretary of Defense, Robert McNamara, who implemented policies he later described as "terribly wrong" and full of "serious misjudgments."

That's why 58,000 Americans (many of them teenage boys) and 3,000,000 Vietnamese (most of them teenage boys) died. My brother-in-law, John, was in the jungles of Vietnam as a seventeen-year-old U.S. Marine. Luckily he, and my cousin Brian, a Marine Officer, made it out alive. U.S. involvement in Vietnam was based on a hidden political agenda rather than clearly defined national objectives—and we paid dearly for it. But as a nineteen year old about to join the military, what the hell did I know—or care—about social consciousness?

After I signed the dotted line to my Navy enlistment, I was ordered to attend a massive military group physical conducted in Newark, New Jersey. It was here that I began to have second thoughts.

My misgivings started when a gruff nurse told me that I had a rare blood type, B negative. I couldn't have been more surprised. "Why," I thought naively, "should my blood type be negative when there were so many positive things in my life?" I quickly learned that this physical wasn't one of the positive things.

I was ushered into a room with fifty other seventeen-to-thirty-year-old guys of every possible size, color, shape and smell, and told to skip down the hall bare-assed naked. "They've got to be kidding me!" I thought to myself as I followed my first of a long list of inane military orders. My second direct order was to do naked jumping jacks while doctors and nurses continued to evaluate our balance and coordination.

I figured this might be a good story for a book someday. Then I thought of a line from one of Shakespeare's plays, "A tale by an idiot, full of sound and fury, signifying nothing." So I changed my mind.

"Welcome to the Navy!" a salty old Chief Petty Officer barked out to us, and the "medical professionals" laughed their asses off at this new shipment of fools. The worst was not over. The grand finale had now just begun.

All fifty of us were ordered by the head nurse—who looked like a fire hydrant in an dirty uniform—to "Bend over, spread your legs, and grab your ankles, NOW!" Then the infamous "Doctor Proctor" quickly went eye-to-asshole with each and every one of us providing the utmost in quality bedside manner and individualized care. It was incredibly humiliating, especially in front of the younger, more attractive nurses. If anything was going to humble me it would be this enlistment. The guy in front of me passed—in both ways—much to the displeasure of the examining physician. It was so pathetic, I was so pathetic, I laughed hysterically. Suddenly I realized that I was the last swingin' dick in line—with all the other swingin' dicks eyeballing me. I remember praying to myself, "Lord, please don't flunk me...not here in front of all of these other assholes."

WHAM!
Guard Dog Neuters Goss

Around the time of my military physical I had been seeing Linda Penney, who was of Russian Jewish heritage. She wore tank tops and platform shoes that raised her small frame about eight inches and drove both the men and the women in my family wild (for differing reasons). We fell easily into a real fun relationship. Her parents treated me great.

I knew Linda's family had a dog named Lance. One evening when I got to her house, Linda answered the door and said, "Bill, my dad's getting tired of putting Lance in the garage every time you come over. He wants to know if you're willing to let the dog get to know you. We think he is probably accustomed to your smell around the house, so there shouldn't be a problem." Even though I was a mere nineteen years old, I already had a wealth of experience with all kinds of animals. I had worked for a veterinarian while in high school. Big dogs weren't a problem for me. Bites in the butt from Boobus's German Shepherd had taught me to move slowly and deliberately around untethered ones. Besides, I was young, fearless and too stupid to know any better. Meeting Lance posed absolutely no danger in my mind. I also assumed the meeting would be carefully supervised by Linda and her father. "Of course I don't mind," I replied.

"Oh, thanks, Bill," Linda's father said. I turned and saw him at the far end of the hallway, his hand resolutely clutching the collar of the biggest, blackest Doberman pinscher I had ever seen. Lance stood over three feet tall at the shoulders and his head was huge. He was as wide at the ears as a dinner plate and had a snout as long as a butcher knife. Still, Lance had a friendly, almost benevolent look in his eyes when Linda's father released his hold.

Lance gingerly trotted up the hall toward me. I stood quietly, without moving, as he sniffed my toes, then my ankles, then my knees, then my crotch. Suddenly and without warning, CHOMP! Lance clamped his jaws over my entire private area. I was stunned. His nose reached my belly button and I could feel the sharpness of his teeth on the cheeks of my ass. I was helpless. I had been "Cujoed." Lance figured it was time for me to pay the devil his due for all the fun I'd had with his master's daughter. Lance growled and tightened his hold on me. He began to back down the hallway, dragging me along by that part of me I thought most important. I mean, I could live without a brain...I had already established that...but I couldn't live without my guy. Believe me, wherever Lance went, I was going. My arms were out to my sides and up in surrender and my eyes must have been getting pretty bulgy as I was pulled along. Lance's eyes were narrowing into slits, getting meaner looking with every backward step he took. The expression "It's a dog eat dog world" suddenly took on a whole new meaning. Linda had her hand to her mouth in horror and her father, who recently had open-heart surgery, fell back against the wall and clutched at his chest.

"What a lawsuit this was going to be..." he probably imagined. Lance, unrelenting, kept backing down the hall, giving my crotch a tooth massage that I'd like to forget.

He led me by the crotch into the den, where Linda's nice mom was intently watching TV. As my buddy Lance and I approached the end of the sofa, I made a muffled plea to her. Linda and her father were still frozen in the hallway. Mrs. Penney looked up, then reacted in horror at the sight. "Oh, my God!" she screamed and instinctively brought her left hand down sharply on Lance's nose. The blow must have hurt like hell because he released me instantly and ran to the corner of the room emitting a demonic and otherworldly sound. He leaped straight up, hitting his head on the ceiling—once, twice, three times—and that was enough for me. I bolted out the door and ran across four lanes of heavy traffic without looking or slowing down. I hoped and prayed that if Lance was at my heels, a Mack truck would flatten either him, or me.

When Linda caught up with me, I told her I didn't think my first meeting with Lance went too well. I also told her they'd better get rid of that dog. The animal was definitely dangerous and unpredictable. The Penneys were attached to Lance though, and couldn't really accept what I said. They wanted to give him another chance. "Another chance at what?" I wondered. As it turned out, my misgivings were correct. The next day Lance attacked Mrs. Penney and shredded her left arm like it had gone through a Vegematic. Then they decided to get rid of him. And that was my last dance with Lance.

About six months after he enlisted, I could tell Bill no longer thought of his earlier girlfriend romantically, but had added her to his list of pals instead. He told me what she had written to him, "I've loved you all the way through, but you're so far away, and we are going on completely different paths now. We'll both change a little, but we'll always have the happy memories of the times we had together. I'd like to think you'll be more than a dusty picture in my wallet eight months from now." She had left the door open, but he had not re-entered. I was secretly glad, but for the life of me, I didn't understand why. We were, after all, just friends.

One of the things I did before leaving for bootcamp was sell my piss-green Volvo Amazon. A guy offered me five hundred bucks for it. What a deal! I figured the Navy would take care of most of my travel arrangements. The day after I sold it, I woke up committed to buying another Amazon when the opportunity arose, but this time it would be mint—no more piss-green colors and caved-in driver's door for me. I started thinking about how to save some money for it as I boarded a military bus in Newark for the twenty-hour trip to Basic Training.

Getting off that bus in Orlando, we must have all looked like outcasts from a rock concert rather than fine, upstanding Navy recruits. Most of us still had long hair and bad attitudes.

We lost both almost immediately. It was a humbling experience, starting with having my healthy head of hair shorn to the scalp. I wondered more than once why I had decided to subject myself to such abuse. It was one of the first times I remember ever doubting a major decision I had made.

I discovered that the race and drug problems in the Navy at the time were pretty damn serious. Boot Camp was mentally demanding, physically grueling and emotionally challenging. It was especially difficult at Christmas time when my mother called to tell me that a very close family friend, a neighbor who had been mugged for eighty-three cents, jumped twenty stories to her death after suffering from chronic depression. I took that news pretty hard. She was a wonderful woman and like a second mother to me.

Like most of the new recruits in my company, I survived the nine weeks of basic training in Orlando. This was in spite of our Company Commander, a second class petty officer who had been busted three times. He was a real dingbat...and a crook...and a con artist. Seeing him in action reminded me that I would be responsible for providing myself the broad education I hoped to get out of my military experience. Though not particularly religious, I made a commitment to read every word of the Bible over the course of the next two years.

After graduating Boot Camp I went to Mineman School in Charleston, South Carolina, to learn how to build underwater bombs. Not many in my class made it through. At times it was pretty tough, though it never occurred to me to give up, or that I might not make it. So I graduated and became a member of MOMAG, which stood for Mobile Mine Assembly Group.

I was given two year orders to a MOMAG detachment in Long Beach, California, where my first official duty was to clean the cage of the detachment's mascot, Alfred E. Gator, or "Al" for short. Assigning the "new kid on the block" with the job of cleaning the alligator pit was the standard initiation, which most guys hated. But I, of course, loved it.

California proved to be a great social set up for me because

I had a buddy, Greg Kay from the University of Arizona, who now lived in Long Beach. He immediately got me connected with the locals. They loved the crude bumper stickers I got for them. Slogans like "Minemen Do It Deeper" or "Minemen Do It With A Bang" were the most popular. Political correctness had not yet taken hold of the U.S. Navy.

When I got to California I bought another Volvo Amazon with the money I had saved. This one was black and I bought it from an Iranian guy who was in a desperate rush to leave the United States for reasons I never learned. It cost one thousand dollars, but it was in mint condition. I loved it.

WHAM!
Goss Sucked Through Jet Engine!

While in Long Beach, I was sent on a special assignment to go aboard the aircraft carrier USS Ranger for three weeks. It was another new adventure for me and I was delighted. I had never been on a military ship before and I knew absolutely zilch about Navy airplanes. I was clueless. I learned shortly that clueless on an aircraft carrier flight deck can nearly be deadly.

I built complete 2000 pound bomb packages beneath the enlisted galley of the ship, which was always crowded and very noisy. I prepared practice Mark 55 and destructor mines for airborne delivery from A-6 Intruders and A-7 Corsairs, Navy jet bombers, that, at the time, I knew nothing about. After attaching the parachute packs on the giant Mark 55s and hooking up the snake-eye speed retardant fins to the smaller, deadlier destructor mines, I used the bomb elevator to take them up to the flight deck. When I surfaced from the bowels of the ship into the blue sky, my ears were bombarded by the sounds of freedom as phantom jets in afterburner rocketed off the forward catapult. Jet blast was everywhere as pilots added power to taxi and turn their aircraft. Giant super thick panels of steel called JBDs or jet blast deflectors went up and down, synchronous with the relative danger of the fifty foot torch coming from the brand new F-14 Tomcats and the much older F-4 Phantom jets. To the hundreds of experienced flight deck personnel who were skillfully, knowledgeably and safely working on the world's most dangerous four acre piece of floating real estate, it was business as usual. Of the hundreds up there who knew what the hell was going on, there was at least one who didn't—me.

My task was to run the arming wires from the parachutes and snake-eye fins to the locking points underneath the wings of the jets. Although this was a simple task, I kept getting blown and sucked across the flight deck by those damn jets. One time, I was knocked down by the blast of a turning F-14 Tomcat. Then it started to blow me towards the huge, very low slung jet intake of an A-7 Corsair. As I held onto a tie-down point on the flight deck to keep from getting sucked into the huge jet engine, the safety officer, a hefty white and green-shirted Lieutenant Commander, signaled to the A-7 pilot to reduce power on his engine. Simultaneously he tackled me and screamed into my thick plastic ear protectors.

At the top of his lungs he yelled, "Son, do you know what they call those things?"

He pointed down the deep, three-foot diameter hole that provides all the oxygen to the huge single engine jet that had moved within ten feet of my flattened position. I shook my head no.

"MAN-EATERS!!!" he screamed again as loudly as he could into my ear protectors.

He then led me to a less deafening part of the aircraft carrier and explained how, in a split second, I could be sucked down the intake of one end of an A-7 only to come out as greasy human hamburger from the exhaust side. I was shown some very graphic photographs of just such things happening. The point was made—very quickly.

I got an extensive lecture on flight deck safety, which the ship had inadvertently neglected to provide me when I checked on board. I never again got on the bad side of an operating jet engine—which I learned was both ends.

After that shipboard adventure, I longed for more adventure, so I requested a transfer back to Charleston, South Carolina. After all, I joined the Navy to see the world, not get stuck in CONUS, military lingo for the "Continental United States." I knew I'd have a better chance to get overseas from Charleston. There was a giant of a man, even bigger than Boobus, named Chief Warrant Officer Petrie, in charge of the Long Beach mine shop. He told me he could arrange the transfer if I could find someone willing to swap with me and not cost the Navy anything. It didn't take long. I got the transfer and soon was driving from Long Beach to Charleston while simultaneously my replacement was driving from Charleston to Long Beach. But my first stop was my hometown of Millburn, New Jersey. I had a full month of Christmas leave before reporting to my new assignment.

Linda and I had parted ways, and that month at home was when I began to really fall for Peggy. There was electricity between us. I had been drawn to her even though our only contact over the past six months had been through the mail. She seemed to sense that it was over between Linda and me. I never said anything, but I could tell she knew. She was more open and relaxed. It was as if there were no more obstacles to the natural progression of our relationship except, of course, the Navy. We had a fabulous month together, and she promised to visit me in South Carolina.

Once in Charleston, I was immediately selected for an overseas assignment to the Mediterranean. I couldn't wait to see Europe. My Commanding Officer sent me on a six-month deployment to Sigonella, Sicily. There I got the opportunity to travel and scuba dive throughout Italy and the island country of Malta. I also climbed to the top of Europe's largest active volcano, 11,000-foot Mt. Etna, and peered into its enormous crater as 4000 degree lava flowed between two rocks where I was standing. As I reflect on that now it was a pretty damn stupid thing to do unless you were gonna fry hamburgers.

As a travel agent, my mother was always checking around

for free and reduced rate trips for my father and her. She worked out a great deal to Italy. I flew to Rome and met them at the Excelsior Hotel, a magnificent hotel where American travel agents were allowed to stay for practically free. I remember awakening in the middle of the first night while on a cot in my parents' room on the tenth floor of this gigantic hotel. I suddenly felt really nauseous, like I was about to get violently seasick. I'll never forget the feeling, it made me want to die. The walls and floor of the hotel vibrated. It reminded me of when the furnace kicked on in our old house in Millburn, and somehow I thought the same thing must happen in this giant 500-room hotel. A minute or two later, the "furnace" kicked off and I was able to get back to sleep. I'll never forget the jolt I got when I saw the headlines on the morning paper they delivered to our room. It read, "Deadly Quake Kills Thousands in N.E. Italy."

Later, I flew to Munich. After assisting an attractive Houston girl with exchanging dollars into marks, I was invited to ride along with her bus group as they toured Southern Germany. She had asked the tour director and he said he wouldn't mind if a U.S. sailor rode for free for a few days. The next morning, I got on the luxury tour bus and what a surprise. The bus was loaded with 26 rich southern belles from colleges in Texas, Georgia, Florida, and Alabama. The only other male on the bus was the 78-year-old tour director. He winked at me when he told me that sixty years earlier he had been a sailor too. It proved to be a fantastic couple of days. But there was a sobering moment, too. While touring Bavaria with these girls, I visited Dachau, Hitler's Jewish extermination camp. It shook my soul to walk through the crematorium knowing that just a generation earlier, millions of innocent men, women and children were tortured, starved, shorn of their hair, and some of their skin. They were more brutally slaughtered than cattle simply because one man didn't like their heritage—and that man was in complete and total control. A trip into Dachau will convince anyone that a voting republic has infinitely better controls incorporated for the good of the people than does fascism or a dictatorship.

Back at work, I used my talents toward putting together underwater bombs and explosives—big ones. It was tense, but satisfying work. At the mineshop in Sigonella, Sicily, we had a mascot, a big friendly dog named Clyde. Every evening we would fill Clyde's enormous food bowl with dry dog food and every morning it would be completely empty. Yet it was bizarre—the dog would be famished, eating every doughnut and omelet we'd smuggle out of the mess hall. I finally figured out that something must be eating his food. So, one day when I had duty and had to spend the night at our remote mineshop location, I hid out of sight and waited to see what animal might come along to steal Clyde's food. Well, after about fifteen minutes of total silence an enormous brown rat appeared from out of nowhere, stuck his head into Clyde's food bowl and started filling his cheeks. Then another, then another. Soon a whole army of monstrous rats was emptying the dog food bowl at an incredibly fast rate. No wonder Clyde was so hungry every morning—he never got a chance to touch his food.

Well, after I told my fellow mineman what I had seen, we immediately dubbed ourselves "The Rat Patrol" and set to work planning their demise. We hooked a 200 pound per square inch pressurized air hose to a blowgun, really more like a blow cannon, which we made out of an eight foot iron pipe. We then made darts out of tenpenny nails and heavy duct tape. It required two men to operate it—one man to pinch the pressurized hose in half, like stopping water in a garden hose, and the other to aim what we dubbed the "Rat Bazooka." Oh, it was ugly to see what this thing could do to a rodent—but you can just imagine. Overnight duty at the mineshop became very popular until all the rats were killed and Clyde was able to eat in peace. The Rat Bazooka was just one of a thousand different kinds of sailor ingenuity I learned as an enlisted man, but it was probably the most memorable.

Now a mineman and not a miner, I enjoyed the thrill of working on some of the world's biggest cherry bombs, designed to crack submarines and battleships in two. I saw classified film footage of their destructive capabilities. What a 2000-pound mine can do to a battleship is truly unbelievable. It literally lifts the ship out of the water and breaks it cleanly in two. If Rat and the Gabers could only see me now!

WHAM!
Blown Tire Destroys Sicilian Town

I remember one particular day that started out pretty much like any other, but it certainly didn't end that way. Mineman First Class Frenchie Fontaine and I were moving mines from one weapons magazine to another, over rutted dirt roads. It had rained for several days, causing more than the usual difficulty for the cumbersome truck I was driving. Loaded on the flatbed were eight of the biggest, meanest non-nuclear weapons the Navy had—2000-pound Mark 55 underwater mines as large as two 55-gallon drums end-to-end. They were loaded with HBX-3, an explosive with three times the explosive power of TNT, and were packed in heavy steel casings. The two-pound boosters of more highly reactive explosives were also installed, but Frenchie and I had ensured that the detonators had been removed. The detonators were loaded with a small but highly reactive explosive called tetryl nitrate which served the equivalent purpose as blasting caps had when I worked in the mines. We didn't take our responsibilities lightly that day, but maybe we should have taken them a little more seriously.

I suppose if there had been time to think I would have been scared to death when the tire blew. But it all happened so fast that I only had time to throw my coffee cup out the window and grab the wheel with both hands. Suddenly the truck took a crazy lurch off the road, tossing the 2000-pound bombs off its flatbed. Frenchie was praying and cursing simultaneously as the huge green bombs bounced off the ground with an unnerving "THEEWWAACK, THEEWWAACK, THEEWWAACK," skipping and skidding along the broken pavement. He believed, with good reason, that the volatile boosters would probably ignite the main charges, rendering us into tiny, unrecognizable bits of flesh and bone scattered like clam sauce over linguini across the Italian countryside. I, on the other hand, was struggling with the steering wheel, just trying to keep the truck upright, cringing as I watched in the sideview mirror the giant bombs tumble and bounce, end over end across the concrete roadway, sparking from the friction. With a final "PAWAANG!" they mercifully buried themselves deep in a muddy embankment.

While watching this whole thing in the truck's mirror, I was determined to keep the grossly imbalanced truck upright. I really had to fight the impulse to close my eyes and cover my ears like the idiot minesweeper timidly tapping the ground in front of him with his feet, prepared for imminent detonation. But, if Frenchie and I were going to die, I didn't want to be the one responsible. It would embarrass my family. As I held on tight to the steering wheel while struggling with the unbalanced truck, my mind raced forward with a myriad of ridiculous thoughts, such as "A mine is a terrible thing to waste" or "The next bomb you drop could be your last."

When the truck finally came to a stop, still upright and somewhat off the road, I turned to assess the battle damage. I looked at those mines being in deep mud as a metaphor of me being in deep shit. But that mud had saved our lives as the bombs found a soft cushion to absorb their most stupendous bounces. The big green mines were covered with muck and slime. Frenchie shook his head and crossed himself, and I'm not ashamed to say I did the same. He then looked at me and said, in his characteristically understated way, "Goss, get the fork lift. Coffee break's over."

We managed to reload the truck and continued on our mission, though we were hours late in our delivery. The junior petty officer who greeted us looked askance at the mud on the weapons, the truck and our uniforms.

"What happened?" he asked with a look of total amazement on his face.

Frenchie looked at him, stoically. "I believe I outrank you son, so don't ask that question again. And it might be wise not to say anything at all."

"Yes, sir," came the reply. It was all I could do to keep from laughing. We could have been in a helluva lot of trouble just about then, or we could have been dead. Instead we were headed for a beer. Frenchie Fontaine drank a helluva lot of beer. I often wondered if I drove him to drink. One time I told him that I thought he drank too much.

"I know my limits," he replied, "I just get drunk before I reach 'em."

Things began to take a more romantic turn for us after Bill came back to New Jersey for a month of Christmas leave prior to his transfer back to Charleston, South Carolina. There had been another girl involved with him for a while, but he broke up with her soon after some crazy dog incident and began to spend all his free time with me. He was fun to be with and I saw a sensitive side to him once or twice that stirred feelings in me that I hadn't felt before. We started having glorious times together.

When Bill got back to Charleston he requested an overseas assignment in his quest to see the world. It was not long in coming. Soon he was a leading seaman, working at a weapons depot in Italy, building underwater bombs in underground ammunition depots. His letters to me, and mine to him, became more and more frequent. Then one day my heart practically leaped out of my chest when I finished reading one of his letters. He had signed it, "I love you."

After six months in Italy, I flew home to meet Peggy in New

York City. We only had a few hours together before I had to catch my connection to Charleston. We wanted some privacy, quickly and badly. We found it in the middle of a junkyard in Jamaica Bay, Queens. Seeing her was like opening presents on Christmas morning. I felt a rush of excitement, joy, anticipation and curiosity. Her face mirrored what I felt, and I knew she was the only woman for me. What a woman! What a junkyard!

Not long after I returned to Charleston Naval Base, I went to the MOMAG Master Chief to follow up on a conversation we had in Sicily. I distinctly remembered him telling me he would get me to Scotland, which was where I wanted to finish my time in the Navy. Then I'd get discharged from the Navy and finish my undergraduate degree with the help of the G.I. Bill.

I walked into his office. "Well, Goss?" he said, "What can I do for you?"

"Scotland, Master Chief," I answered. "You said you'd get me there."

This time he had a decidedly less friendly look as I reminded him of his earlier promise to me. Sarcastically, he replied, "You're a short timer, Goss. You've only got about a year to go. There is no way I'm going to cut you a set of cherry orders like Scotland. We'll come up with something else for you to do."

I was too angry to answer. He had given me his word in Italy, had made it sound like a given that I would get deployed to Scotland. I had been looking forward to living in Great Britain for months.

"Yes, Master Chief," I said, gritting my teeth. I got up and walked out. Blinded with anger, I stepped out of his office and smack into a monster of a man, Lieutenant Petrie. I stepped back and respectfully apologized, as befitting a junior enlisted sailor. Then I recognized him as my old Officer in Charge from Long Beach, the one who had arranged my transfer back to Charleston. He had received a big promotion—probably for getting me out of California—and also a transfer. I'd heard he'd been killed in a wild car accident in his corvette. He greeted me warmly, and I told him of my anger and disappointment after my conversation with the Master Chief.

"Well, Mineman Goss," he said, "I think you should volunteer to be the Admiral's driver."

I looked at him in amazement. Rear Admiral Duffy had the reputation of being the meanest, toughest short man on earth. Bulldogs ran from him. He was known as "The Human Hand Grenade With Legs" by his staff.

"I don't think so," I replied.

"No, I'm serious Seaman Goss, I really think you should volunteer to be the Admiral's driver," he repeated, his twinkling, eyes peering into mine. He gave no explanation for his statement, simply repeated it with the same, decided conviction.

Blinking, I said, "I'll think about it." And I did. I thought about it all night long and concluded that just maybe, in a weird way, God had selected Lt. Petrie to be one of my guardian angels.

The next day, I went back to the Command Master Chief and volunteered to be the Admiral's river. Apparently, no one else wanted the job, or maybe the Master Chief thought he would punish me by calling his hand on Scotland, because in no time at all he had me in my new assignment as Admiral's Driver.

Everything I had heard was true. The man was meaner than a rabid wildcat with hemorrhoids. He habitually tore into his subordinates, especially his "Four Stripers," the full Navy captains under his command. He'd have me sit outside his door, intentionally left open, to further humiliate them. Sometimes he'd rant as if he was stark raving crazy while standing on the top of his large, glass covered desk. Only then could he look down at them as they stood quivering at attention. One Captain with a severe stutter was brought to tears by one of the Admiral's unrelenting tirades. It was a most unusual management technique. Somehow Admiral Duffy had confused the last word in the acronym "MBO" which stands for "Management By Objectives," with either "Oppression" or "Omnipotence." The whole experience was very motivating because I knew I had the potential to do a better job than this. A seed in the back of my brain began to germinate.

Long ago all naval officers wore black shoes with all their uniforms. When airplanes were introduced to the Navy, naval aviators started wearing brown shoes to set themselves apart from the less highly regarded ship drivers. This naval aviation tradition continues to irritate the non-flyboy type naval officers to this day. They have argued, to deaf ears thankfully, for a return to a one-shoe color Navy. Someday, I, too, would become a commissioned officer. And not only that, but I would "one up" Admiral Duffy. I wouldn't be a "Blackshoe" like him. I'd be a "Brownshoe."

As tough as the Admiral was to work for, he was always fair to me, and I liked him. I used to drive his jet black sedan, with his two star flag flying on the front, up to the airport to pick up Peggy when she came down to visit. Peggy would see sailors snap to attention and salute us as we drove through the gates of the Charleston Navy Base.

"You must be important," Peggy once commented.

"Yeah, Seaman Goss is reaaallllly important," I chuckled to myself. I'm sure the Admiral knew I didn't bother to take his flag down when I drove to pick her up. The thought probably made him laugh. For some unknown reason, he seemed to like me. He let me get away with things that a higher-ranking sailor would have suffered an ugly death over. In fact, the Admiral even seemed a bit protective of me.

I'll never forget what he did the night of my first boxing competition on his base. It was what we called a "smoker." The boxing ring was outside and surrounded by bleachers crowded with loud, opinionated sailors, and several fellow minemen. My opponent was a tough, very muscular street brawler with limited boxing skills. I was literally destroying him when he bent his head down and blindly charged toward me. Frustrated from not being able to land a punch, he was going to butt me, and my reaction was instinctive. I pushed his head down and away with my right and gave him an uppercut as hard as I could with my left. Because of the way he charged me with his face down, it was an almost unavoidable violation on my part if I was to defend myself at all. It happened three times, and each time I defended myself from his idiotic charge toward me in the same way. I thought I had an easy victory, but much to my chagrin the scoring referees awarded my opponent five punches for each of my fouls, and took away five scoring blows from me. It's not like I tried to bite off his ear....

Even with that grotesque point spread, the decision was split. Two of the three referees declared my opponent the winner because of the violations, and when the referee raised my opponent's hand to signify his victory, the crowd went wild in disbelief. Boos and hisses arose from all corners of the arena. Then a short figure in a starched white uniform climbed into the ring and shook my hand. On each shoulder board was a thick gold stripe and two gold stars. It was Admiral Duffy, all five foot two inches of him.

The Admiral, still in great shape, had been a varsity fighter at Notre Dame where he earned a master's degree in chemistry. He began to shout at the referees, reducing them to nothing more than dog meat. I was extremely embarrassed, and also oddly pleased. What he did was totally against any protocol I had ever learned, but he did it for me. He made a hit with the sailors that day because he was right. I clearly beat the tar out of that guy and he wasn't going to let a couple of two-bit referees tell him any different.

A few months later, the Navy, still suffering from the Z-Grams of the former CNO Admiral Elmo Zumwalt, eliminated the position of Admiral's driver altogether. They decided admirals weren't quite important enough to have full time drivers.

"Sorry, Bill," he said. "I don't have a choice. I've got to let you go. You'll be going back to your old command, MOMAG."

I'm sure he could tell I didn't want to be back under the supervision of the Master Chief that had lied to me.

"What would you like to do?" the Admiral asked.

"I'd really like to go to Scotland," I answered.

He smiled. "I think maybe you'll get there," was all he said.

Later when I walked into the Master Chief's office, he motioned me into a chair.

"Well..." he trailed off.

"I'd like to fly home to New Jersey to spend Thanksgiving with my girlfriend and my family. Then I'd like to fly from there to Scotland," I said boldly.

"You can pick up your plane tickets tomorrow," was all he said.

"In the middle of difficulty lies opportunity."
—Albert Einstein

"No woman ever falls in love with a man,
unless she has a better opinion
of him than he deserves."
—Author Unknown

CHAPTER FOUR

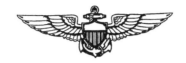

THE NEWLYWED GAME

L iving in the highlands of Scotland above Loch Lomond was all I thought it would be. The perfect finish for my Navy stint. I spent every weekend hitchhiking throughout Great Britain, exploring the nooks and crannies, visiting all the out-of-the-way and unusual places. My letters to Peggy described everything, and I felt closer to her than ever. "I feel like I'm on the mailing list for your mother's travel agency." She wrote, "Your postcards and letters are wonderful. Inverness Castle is so beautiful, I must see it!" She didn't know she had, for I had felt her presence beside me. Exploring all over Scotland, England, Wales and the outlying islands, then getting out of the Navy and coming home to Peggy would really be a dream come true.

WHAM!
Shotgun Blast Parts Hair

My two-year active duty commitment was just about up and I flew from Scotland to Charleston to prepare for the transition back to civilian life. During this time I visited with Barney Hunt, a backwoods son of a dairy farmer and a former mineman classmate of mine who lived an hour north of Charleston. Unfortunately, Barney had flunked out of mineman school and the Navy decided not to retain him in the military service, a very atypical but intelligent decision on their part. Instead, the Navy sent Barney back to the farm before he "bought the farm." Evidently, in the Navy's infinite wisdom, they viewed him as a real hazard around "things that go BANG." We continued our friendship largely because Barney and his family were wonderfully kindhearted farm folk who generously invited me to visit with them whenever I was not overseas. The huge dairy barn was snake heaven. In it, I ended up catching my next college roommate, Petey, a giant seven-foot black ratsnake, a friendly critter like the one Rat caught when we were kids. Petey stayed with me for years.

Now, Barney was a good ole boy who did a little poaching once in a while. He had somehow managed to have his new double barrel shotgun confiscated a few days before I came up to visit. When I arrived, Barney persuaded me to try to talk the game warden into returning his gun. Knowing I'd have a better shot with the warden than Barney would, I did just that. It was that same gun, later that afternoon that almost killed me.

The two of us had been sitting at the kitchen table. Barney had been drinking beer and some of Orangeburg's famous killer moonshine (which really killed a whole party of people one summer), while I had been getting ready for the hour drive back to Charleston. Barney decided to give me a shooting demonstration with his newly returned weapon. As Barney and I, walking side by side, took that first step out his door and onto his front porch, he released the gun's safety and KAABBOOOOMMM! Both barrels exploded just below my left ear. I felt blast and shot graze through my hair and looked up to see a gaping, smoking hole blown right through the roof of the porch. Barney Hunt, totally shocked and distraught, sat down on the porch steps, trembling. I would have joined him, but at the time I was suddenly overcome by an urge to get out of town.

"Thanks for the demonstration, Barney, but next time I'll take a rain check," I said, rather disconcerted. I jumped in the Amazon for the drive back to Charleston. I didn't get the shakes until I was about twenty miles down the road. I felt gunpowder burns in my scalp while running my fingers through my hair. What would the top of my head have looked like if that gun's barrel had been pointed three quarters of an inch lower? I remembered the words of my foreman in the copper mines. Yes, I was one lucky Blond Chiquita and this time I had just narrowly escaped being scalped with a shotgun by a good buddy. It was my last visit to Orangeburg and the last time I've ever hung around anyone who had a gun, a six pack, and a penchant for messing with them at the same time. Call me crazy.

I received an honorable discharge from the Navy and used the G.I. Bill and a tuition grant to attend Rutgers University. There, in my spare time, I trained and fought in the New Jersey Golden Gloves. Generally I studied hard, courted Peggy and played it safe. I stayed in the Navy Reserve and continued to use my military training by working weekends on underwater explosives at the Navy Weapons Depot in Earle, New Jersey.

One particularly fascinating course at Rutgers was in the Communications and Media Department. It was called "Persuasion" and was a study in the dynamics between the Persuader and the Persuadee, a word not found in the dictionary because I just made it up. For my class project, I joined forces with another student in the class, Nina Docker. We devised an experiment where we would find women who were deathly afraid of snakes and within five minutes (timed on a hidden stopwatch) I would have them holding "Tut," a five-foot long nonpoisonous kingsnake. Although, of course, there would be no way of them knowing whether it was poisonous or not. That was the persuading part of the study. Neither Nina nor I had ever seen or met any of these college women before, but we got all ten women to let Nina and me, total strangers, invite ourselves into their dormitory room at night, even when they were completely alone. We had all ten of these coeds holding a five-foot long snake within a few minutes. To verify this, we took photos of all of them holding Tut with pained, horrified expressions on their faces. In that regard, the study was a great success. But speaking of snakes, the male professor gave Nina, who was rather attractive, an "A" on the project and gave me a "B+" even though I had planned and organized the entire experiment. All Nina had done was to gather the data. I guess I should have put more effort into persuading the professor and less effort into persuading the coeds. Oh well.

I learned three things from this experiment:

1) Artful persuasion is an extremely powerful tool, capable of conquering people's worst fears in mere minutes.
2) College coeds are too trusting of complete strangers, especially when they are alone at night.
3) When your professor is a snake, it pays to be a good-looking coed rather than a creative guy.

The summer of my junior and winter of my senior years, I spent a total of sixteen weeks in Pensacola, Florida, attending Aviation Officer Candidate School. Initially, I had been toying with the idea of becoming a Navy pilot. Gunnery Sergeant Buck Welcher and Staff Sergeant Cleveland of the United States Marine Corp taught me an important lesson during those two challenging eight week training programs— don't toy with anything, just do it. The harder they made it, the more I wanted it. Even with the lack of sleep, challenging academics, constant abuse to convince the less committed officer candidates to DOR (Drop on Request), the physical training in "The Rose Garden," surprise room and locker inspections called "Hurricanes," the pressure chamber, survival and parachute training, the "Dilbert Dunker" and the helo crash simulators at water survival. It was time to begin a career, and a career as a Navy pilot—if they'd have me— seemed like a dream job come true. I'd "just do it" no matter how tough the program. My tour as the Admiral's driver had inspired me not to go back into the Navy unless I was a commissioned officer. I also felt confident that I could do a better job as a naval officer than some I had observed. Admiral Duffy, unwittingly, had taught me how not to lead.

After Bill got out of the Navy and was accepted into Rutgers, he rented a house with three other bachelors. I was living near Kean College, the school I attended, with three single women. Bill and I saw each other whenever we weren't working at our part-time jobs or cramming for exams. It was a fun time with not much sleep.

Bill had never expressed an interest in going back into the Navy until I bought him a single engine airplane introductory flight for his 23rd birthday at Morristown Municipal Airport. The next thing I knew he announced that he was accepted into the Navy's flight program, with a guarantee of becoming a student pilot candidate if he passed a sixteen-week officer candidate school in Pensacola, Florida. He made it sound like it would be easy, but I had my doubts.

I never thought that a little flight in a Cessna for fifteen minutes could change someone's life so dramatically, but it did—both mine and his, in extraordinary ways.

This period at Rutgers was different for Bill than at University of Arizona. He kept his hair much shorter and didn't have to nearly kill himself to make ends meet. We studied hard, worked hard and dated hard, but not necessarily in that order. Bill was very excited about becoming a Navy pilot. He worked like crazy to finish his studies in economics and ecology so he could get back to Pensacola and complete the last eight weeks of the officer commissioning program. He ran and worked out so that he'd be in top shape for the physical side of the program, which evidently was quite intense.

I was working hard to complete my degree in English and business administration and couldn't wait to spend my waitress earnings touring Europe with my friend Bonnie. Thoughts of marriage never crossed my mind, especially after Bill announced he was going into the Navy again. I didn't think either of us were ready yet for that kind of commitment—marriage or the Navy.

I was in a rush to become a Navy pilot. I had always wanted to fly, but could never afford it. Just being a military officer seemed like a big deal to me—Kennedy, Johnson, Nixon, Ford, Carter, they had all been naval officers. I wanted to be a Navy pilot like George Bush, receive the multi-million dollar flight training and maybe follow it all up with a career as an airline pilot. I was inspired by a quote from Charles Lindbergh, "Science, freedom, beauty, adventure. What more could you ask of life? Aviation combined all the elements I loved."

My greatest motivation was that I wanted to make Peggy and my family proud. If being a U.S. Navy pilot wouldn't make them proud, I thought, nothing would.

I assumed that it would require an enormous amount of concentration and self-discipline to get through the naval aviation program. I knew I was too easily distracted and my memory needed to be improved if I wanted to have a fighting chance of pinning on those coveted Wings of Gold. So, I started one-on-one sessions with Dr. Harry Aaron, a world-renowned expert in self-hypnosis. At his office in New Jersey, he taught me tricks on how to focus and how to memorize, how to relax and how to persevere. He also gave me a break on his fee. What a great guy. When I used his techniques, they never failed me.

I was in so much of a rush to start flight school that I received my commission as a naval officer prior to actually graduating college—which, according to the Navy, was "administratively impossible." I remember when the Navy finally received my diploma, my graduation date was a few months after I had started flight training. I was also questioned as to how I finished with only 119.5 college credits when Rutgers required 120 to graduate. I told them they rounded up. The bureaucracy didn't like my answers. But I didn't like their questions so I figured that made us even.

Shortly after I had returned from my trip to Europe, Bill was getting ready to leave for his final eight weeks of Aviation Officer

Candidate School or AOCS, as he called it. He proposed one night after a candle lit dinner. I accepted and both sets of parents seemed to be pleased. That didn't last long.

A few months later, Bill invited me down to Pensacola to watch his officer commissioning ceremony. It was a really big deal. He was now Ensign Goss, United States Navy. His parents were there and they were very proud, especially his Dad.

I met Bill's Drill Instructor (fondly referred to as a "D.I.") but who Bill only knew as "Gunnery Sergeant Buck Welcher, United States Marine Corps, Sir!" What a character this guy Welcher was. Buck ended up taking two months leave from the Marines to become actor Lou Gossett, Jr.'s technical advisor for the movie An Officer *and a* Gentleman, *which depicts the officer candidate program that Bill completed. Lou Gossett, won the Academy's "Best Actor" award for his portrayal as a Marine D.I., and Bill swears Gossett on the silver screen was the spitting image of Gunny Buck in action.*

This was the third "to the bone" haircut the Navy had given Bill in the five years I'd known him. But, it didn't matter to me if Bill had shoulder length hair or no hair at all. And, it didn't seem to affect him or change his personality one iota. He was both the craziest and sanest person I'd ever met.

I got to Pensacola a week before his graduation. Bill was fighting in the base boxing tournament a few hours after he picked me up at the airport. He must have been pretty excited to see me because he knocked his opponent out cold and they had to carry the poor guy out of the ring. Although I knew he had been a golden-glove boxer in college, it was a side of Bill I had never seen before—that of a real tough guy.

The day after the boxing tournament, we arranged to see the base chaplain about marrying us as soon as possible. The Navy was not very flexible in allowing time off for their future naval aviators, and marriage early in the program was generally discouraged. We met with the chaplain, who was a Catholic priest and senior Navy Captain, and asked him to marry us. I'll never forget his reply. "No, you'll be divorced in less than a year." That single,

*brusque statement inspired Bill and me to keep our marriage to-
gether no matter what. That chaplain may have been quoting per-
centages or odds, but if there is one thing that Bill holds in contempt, it's when people tell him that the odds are not in his favor.
He refuses to look at himself as a statistic, and when other people
do, it actually energizes him.*

*Bill then persuaded me, unbeknownst to our parents, to be
married by the local Justice of the Peace the day after his parents left
Pensacola. He figured that if my parents couldn't be there to see us
marry then neither would his. He's a very fair-minded guy. So a
few days after Bill became Ensign William Allan Goss, United
States Navy, I became Mrs. Margaret Gleason Goss. I also became,
in the eyes of the Navy but unknowingly to me, a "dependent." It's
an insulting term coined by the U.S. Department of Defense and I
have despised it for the past fifteen years. I can't see why the term
"spouse" won't do!*

*On the drive from Pensacola, Florida, to Corpus Christi, Texas,
we called home to tell our parents that we had eloped. The news
was terribly received. Bill's parents were angry and hurt because
they had just been down to see us days before. My parents, on the
other hand, were upset because we didn't get married by a Catholic
priest.*

*The only phone call to New Jersey that was not a disaster was to
Bill's grandparents. Their response was "Oh, that's nice." What I
didn't know at the time was that they had married against their
parents' wishes over sixty years earlier. Bill's grandmother got
married in a bright red flapper dress of the roaring twenties. Their
marriage, too, had been slightly unconventional.*

*We arrived at Naval Air Station Corpus Christi, Texas, after
twelve hours in Bill's unbearably hot 200,000 miles plus Volvo, an
extremely upset and downtrodden young newlywed couple. We were
devastated that everyone was so upset with us and that my poor
new husband had fallen from grace with such a loud, resounding
thud.*

*I, on the other hand, was thrown into a way of life so unfamil-
iar for a suburban New Jersey girl that I was shell-shocked. The*

night after we arrived in Corpus Christi, we went to see a movie at the base theater. We were the only people in the audience. It was The Great Santini *starring Robert Duvall as a naval aviator who destroyed the lives of his wife and children. It was a real crash and burn kind of movie. After the movie was over, Bill and I sat alone on the outside steps, under wildly blowing palm trees against a jet black sky. Feeling incredibly vulnerable, even while in each other's arms, we cried in the darkness. Being a newlywed was supposed to feel a little bit better than this, I thought. Our marriage was off to a rocky start.*

*"One neglects to see an important factor in love, that of will.
To love somebody is not just a strong feeling—
it is a decision, it is a judgment, it is a promise.
If love were only a feeling,
there would be no basis for the promise
to love each other forever.
A feeling comes and it may go.
How can I judge that it will stay forever,
if my actions do not involve judgment and decision?"
—Erich Fromm*

"A pessimist complains God puts thorns on roses,
while an optimist thanks God
He put roses on thorns."
—Author Unknown

CHAPTER FIVE

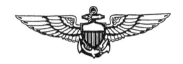

IN THE NAVY: ROUND TWO— AN OFFICER AND A GENTLEMAN

R ight after Peggy and I eloped, I started flight training in the T-28 Trojan. It was a gigantic single-engine carrier-capable airplane with an enormous 1425 horsepower 9-cylinder radial engine. The sound from it was deafening. And, it wasn't air-conditioned. I suffered miserably on my first flight, with a frustrated flight instructor behind me yelling and throwing things while we orbited above Padre Island in the brutally hot Texas sun.

It wasn't much better at home. I had to study and memorize procedures endlessly. As Peggy and I descended from shock into depression at the anger expressed by our parents over our elopement, I suddenly felt the urge to do something utterly foreign to my soul—quit. It certainly appeared to be an easy thing to do as I watched several of my friends quit, even those with lots of prior flight time. They just couldn't take the pressure anymore. I knew I was already past the cracking point. But instead, I prayed the Navy would kick me out so I wouldn't have to quit.

Although I was not an ace student, my problems weren't solely due to my fall from grace with my parents or the accompanying depression. Although most of the instructors were dedicated professionals, a few were real jerks. One particularly obnoxious flight instructor popped positive for cocaine and was caught sleeping with the enlisted girls as well. He wasn't a great role model and all the student pilots were glad to see him get booted out of the Navy.

I got airsick during the first five flights. Whether it was due to the incredible heat and lack of air circulation, massive sensory overload, an inner ear infection, a bad case of the jitters or a combination of all these things, it was torturous. Finally, my instructor recommended my training be stopped. This decision was bittersweet for me, but I tried to accept it and started working with the Navy Supply Department. After a few weeks of learning Inventory Control and Logistics from a salty old Supply Corps Officer, I found myself gazing through his office window watching a helicopter practice autorotations. "Bill, you don't want to be a Supply Officer, you want to be a pilot. What are you doing here?"

"What am I doing here?" I suddenly asked myself.

During my lunch break an hour later, I was knocking on the back door of Commodore Ward's office at his big headquarters. As the senior Navy Captain and Wing Commander, he was responsible for the training of the several hundred student pilots on the base.

"A...a...ah...yes...?" Commodore Ward said, turning in his chair and wondering why an impudent Navy Ensign was poking his head through his private office entrance rather than dealing with his secretary in the traditional manner in the reception room.

"Commodore Ward, I'm Ensign Goss and I need to talk to you." I said in the most respectful and endearing way possible.

He invited me in and patiently listened to my story about my elopement with Peggy and both of our families' big disappointment with us, and how, because of it, airsickness had ended my training. I further explained that I was willing to do anything to get another chance at earning my Navy pilot wings of gold.

The look in his eyes was kind, yet stern. "Ensign Goss, your airsickness is probably because of your apprehension of flying. I flew A-6 Bombers in Vietnam, and I'm here to tell you that a certain amount of apprehension in a pilot is to be appreciated.

Fearlessness certainly is not." On his desk was a plaque that read,

There are old pilots
And there are bold pilots
But there are no old, bold pilots.

"Bill, if you can channel your apprehension and learn to control it, you won't get airsick and you'll earn those Wings of Gold. I'm going to send you to a special one-week program in Pensacola, where aviation physiologists will evaluate your aeronautical adaptability. If they are able to, they will teach you how to overcome your airsickness so that you can become a good Navy pilot. You certainly have a drive and enthusiasm that I wish more of your peers would demonstrate. Good luck. One more thing...next time come in through the front door of my office...understand Ensign Goss?"

"Yes, sir!" I said, standing to shake his hand. "Thank you, Commodore!"

And that is just what happened. I learned new techniques, got over the post-elopement blues, worked through things with my new bride and got acclimated to being upside down in airplanes.

After twelve instructional flights, beg, borrow or steal, I finally "strapped on" this monstrously overpowered airplane and took off alone. Solo. What a rush! Suddenly the whole program made sense to me—to wear out and abuse the students until only the most motivated finished. "And to think how hard it was to get Dad to give me the keys to the car" I thought while dropping into a 350 mph dive over Padre Island. "If Dad could only see me now!" I laughed aloud in my oxygen mask as the massive radial engine begged for more.

I discussed with Peggy what kind of plane I felt would be best for me to fly, and concluded that flying the powerful multi-mission P-3 Orion would be ideal. After primary flight school the student pilot grades are tabulated. Based on those grades and the needs of the Navy, you are selected to fly either props, jets or helos. It's still the ultimate crapshoot for the young Navy student pilots and their families. Typically we had almost no input as to what type aircraft we would be assigned to fly or where in the world we'd end up. One buddy who wanted to fly jets based in California ended up flying helos based in Cuba. But he enjoyed what he got, which also was typical. Fortunately, I got my first choice, P-3s out of Brunswick, Maine. Trust me, good grades had nothing to do with it.

After flying the T-28 Trojan, affectionately nicknamed the "lead sled" by those who walked away unharmed from crashes in farmers fields, I flew 100 hours in the T-44 King Air. This is a much newer twin engined jet prop with state of the art radios and navigation equipment, and thank God, air-conditioning. It was like moving up from a Harley to a Cadillac. And it was easier, so I found the time to train for and win the base boxing smoker in the light-heavy weight division. Peggy and I also took time out to drive the black Volvo Amazon through Northern Mexico, and to visit my Aunt Fran and brother Larry in Houston and Austin.

Soon the day I thought would never come finally arrived—the famous "Winging Ceremony." When Peggy pinned those coveted Navy Pilot Wings of Gold above my left breast pocket in front of my parents and family it was my proudest moment—just incredible.

At first it had seemed like way too much emotional sacrifice until I saw how proud Bill was the day I pinned on his "Navy Wings of Gold." "Finally," I thought, "all this work and sacrifice was worth something." It had been a year since our brutally received elopement. Now the new pilot was grinning from ear to ear. It made me cry to see that once again, in the eyes of his parents, Bill was the prodigal son.

I remember reading an inscription under a set of Navy pilot

wings. It said, "Many may fly and some are rewarded hand-somely, but this emblem means more than flying. It is dearly bought, requires sacrifice to keep, and represents a way of life." I had learned to become one with an airplane. With the constant potential for airborne disaster, nothing is as exhilarating as flying low and fast. High flight, above the clouds, connected with the heavens, is an equally inspiring and totally different experience. The joy of flight is simply sublime.

A few days after getting my Navy pilot wings, Peg and I packed up the old Amazon and made the two-day drive from the "Texas Riveria" to Jacksonville, Florida. There I would begin flight training as a newly designated naval aviator in Lockheed's $60 million aircraft, the P-3 Orion.

With around 20,000 horsepower, a top speed of about 500 mph, and a highly trained twelve-man crew, the Orion was one helluva weapons platform. It could carry torpedoes, mines, conventional weapons and special weapons—a powerful nuclear depth bomb designed to crack the hull of Soviet ballistic missle submarines. It had been said that one of these depth bombs could vaporize a cubic mile of ocean water. The Orion could also launch the harpoon missile, capable of taking out a battle-ship or heavy cruiser from nearly 100 miles and could fly over fourteen hours non-stop. The P-3 Orion was designed to get to trouble spots around the globe quickly, often tracking Soviet submarines without their knowledge and fulfilling a myriad of other valuable functions in the interests of national defense. A superb multi-purpose weapons platform, it was highlighted in Tom Clancy's Cold War thriller, *The Hunt for Red October.*

After completing six more months of advanced flight training in Jacksonville, and winning its boxing light-heavy weight division, I drove up to Brunswick with Peg. We stopped off in New Jersey. There I rented a Grumman Tiger from a TWA pilot at Morristown Airport. A couple hours later, he and I were doing tight circles in the moonlight around the Statue of Liberty, with my delighted parents in the back seat, celebrating their wedding anniversary with a bottle of champagne. I never would have done this on my own but the TWA captain had a lot of nighttime experience flying over Manhattan. He called it his "moonlight madness" flight. My parents thought it was a great wedding anniversary gift and we all had a ball.

Once in Maine, I fulfilled a promise to myself by signing up at a nearby college to start a Master of Business Administration degree program. I also fulfilled a promise to Peg with a tiny black and brown puppy that we named Scooter, an adorable Yorkshire terrier that fit comfortably in one of my black flight boots. Within weeks I was deployed to Bermuda for six months flying spy missions against "Red" submarines, while Peggy and Scooter settled into a comfortable old home we bought in Bath, Maine. It had been built 100 years earlier by a local cigar merchant who kept the area shipbuilders stogied up.

WHAM!
Goss Plane Taken to the Land of Oz

While flying against a particularly stealthy Soviet Victor class attack submarine at dawn in the Bermuda Triangle, our crew navigator and my good buddy, Pat "Bo" Mills, requested we execute a hard right turn back to the turnover sonar buoy. The plane we were relieving had dropped it to help us maintain our position. In the middle of my aggressive turn to the submerged sub's last known location, a tornado, known as a waterspout over the open ocean, came into sight directly in our flight path. I banged a hard turn to the left and yelled back to Bo, "Hey, Navigator, we almost flew into a tornado!"

Bo responded in his usual naive, jovial way, "Get out of town, Wild Bill—the other plane told me that a tornado was over three miles from here. It can't be the same one, you knucklehead, can it?"

"Bo, what am I going to do with you? Tornadoes move all over the place...didn't you see *The Wizard of Oz*?" That evening, Bo and I dressed up as Jake and Elwood of the Blues Brothers, visited the Bermuda Officers' Club—and the drinks were on him, both literally and figuratively.

Bo and I were sent to Iceland on another special mission with our crew. While flying out of Iceland, we would sometimes track billion dollar Soviet ballistic missile subs, called "Typhoons," hiding under the ice north of the Arctic Circle. At night—and wintertime was virtually perpetual night—the light shows in the sky were spectacular. The aurora borealis or Northern lights, as it is commonly known, would shimmer above us like a brilliant translucent veil. That, combined with the stars and meteors that filled the sky, has caused pilots to get vertigo (especially when the ocean beneath them is lit with the lights of fishing boats), and sometimes caused them to fly inverted into the dark ocean below thinking it was the sky above. Flying with unreliable flight instruments and without a visible horizon in the clouds could really be hell on pilots' nerves.

St. Elmo's Fire is another bizarre phenomenon I sometimes encountered in situations where flying very close to thunderstorms was unavoidable. Accurate weather forecasts were virtually impossible to get 1000 miles out in the middle of the ocean. It was a fact of life that never stopped us from attempting to fly the mission. And it was usually on these missions when St. Elmo would come visit for a spell.

Suddenly, while being bounced around in the black storm turbulence—with the red instrument lights just a fuzzy blur as I tried to maintain altitude—fingers of static electricity, like miniature lighting bolts, would creep up and down the aircraft's windshield. If I inadvertently flew even closer to the center of the thunderstorm, the static electricity would enter the cockpit and dance on the instruments, on the power levers and on my hands. It was an enchanting, but deadly sign. For when St. Elmo visits a pilot in the cockpit, that airplane is in imminent danger of being struck by lighting. You have entered into the storm's most dynamic area of static discharge. At times it seemed that it would be a miracle if my crew and I made it through to the other side of the storm without being struck by lightning. Or beaten to death by golf ball sized hail or torrents of rain and snow—

shaking us to pieces like rag dolls in the severe turbulence.

As we often flew twelve-hour missions throughout the night, falling asleep at the wheel was a real possibility. Fatigue is probably the worst thing a pilot has to deal with. Total exhaustion can make you forget the consequences of your actions as you enter into a dream-state. It's happened to most pilots who fly at night. When you open your eyes with a start, it is a terrifying feeling to see right before your eyes the red cockpit lights of the airplane that is supposed to be in your total control. It is almost impossible to get enough sleep before the night flights because forcing oneself to sleep in the middle of the day is hard to do. Although the pilots unanimously dreaded the "all night burners," it's the price we gladly paid for the privilege of flight and for the satisfaction of annotating one's logbook at the end of the week.

WHAM!
Ambiance Kills Goss Couple

The night I got home from my first six-month deployment, Peg and I built a roaring fire in our huge old wood stove as it stormed outside. I remember drinking a bottle of wine with her as we enjoyed each other's company on the sleeper sofa and then we passed out. I awoke with a splitting headache and looking around the wall at the candelabras. I felt upside down—and confused. All the candles were pointing towards the hardwood floor and the air was absolutely stifling, unbreathable. I tried to wake Peggy, but couldn't. When I tried to stand, I collapsed. I crawled on my elbows to a window and struggled to open it. Finally it popped open. The hot carbon monoxide blasted out, and the freezing, sub-zero fresh air blasted in. I dragged Peggy into the hall and we both held our heads in pain. We had consumed a lot of wine but definitely not that much. It turned out that the room had gotten so hot that the many unlit candles on the wall had become softened and caused them to flop down from pointing to the ceiling to pointing to the floor. The huge fire had sucked all the oxygen from that tiny room and almost asphyxiated us. That, my friend, was one of the hottest times Peggy and I ever had!

WHAM!
Goss Saved by Luggage

The following spring I caught a plane on its way to Malmstrom AFB, Montana, with another Navy lieutenant, Brian Mee. We stayed at the Bear Creek Ranch, a big-game hunting camp that backed up to Glacier National Park and was owned and run by my close friends, Doctor "Big Al" Speidell and Billy Beck.

Brian and I spent our first evening there at a cowboy bar teaching the locals how to drink shots of whiskey while standing on our heads. Quite successful in this endeavor, we hobbled back to our cabin in the wee hours of the morning smoking cigarettes, something neither of us normally did—but hell, we'd been drinking.

We threw our cigarettes into the mud in order to pick up our luggage (which had been set outside the cabin door) then we burst through the doorway. The rotten egg smell of propane blasted us in the face as we looked at each other in wonderment and then ran out. We stared at our cigarettes still smoldering on the ground. Evidently the water heater gas line had broken and had been filling the cabin for the past week. If we had walked in there sucking on those cigarettes, we would have instantly flown back to Maine without the luxury of a plane. Brian and I never had the urge to smoke again.

Deep in the snow covered mountains of Northern Maine lies a little known and highly unpopular resort owned by the U.S. Navy called "SERE" School for Survival, Evasion, Rescue and Escape. This enormous tract of land is set up to prepare pilots and aircrew for the POW experience in the event they are shot down over enemy territory. I volunteered to attend it while a very junior lieutenant because attendance was becoming mandatory for military pilots and the more senior your rank the more difficult "the opposing forces" made the experience for you. And what an experience it was. I cannot divulge exactly what goes on during this weeklong school. I can tell you this, parts of it took place deep in a mountain forest in an incredibly convincing prisoner of war camp—at least to the brainwashed trainees. Unbeknownst to us, we were carefully and continually monitored through one-way mirrors by staff psychologists. The SERE School experience left me with an indelible imprint of what my strengths and weaknesses are. I learned how to deal more logically and systematically with personal and group aspects of survival while being interrogated and tortured, naked, in four feet of snow. I discovered that the classic John Wayne-type military man is killed off quickly in such settings to create a workable level of subservience in the prisoner/guard relationship. This also prevents leadership through heroics from being outwardly displayed by the POWs. Through firsthand experience, I learned that brainwashing was in fact a very powerful ability that the enemy would capitalize on. I died many unnecessary deaths at that camp which was exactly what the Navy did not want to happen to their pilots that end up being taken prisoner. When I saw the American flag raised at the end of training, it was a deeply moving experience for us all. It left me with a renewed sense of patriotism and awe at the freedoms many of us routinely take for granted.

At work the following week, a very agitated Peggy called me on the phone. "Bill, the mailman just placed a package on the steps, rang the doorbell and ran like hell."

"Great, Peg, open it up," I said curiously.

"No way, it's covered in blood."

I could tell from the disgust in her voice that I was getting nowhere fast. "Honey, what's the return address?"

"Montana," she replied.

"I'll be home in a minute, dear. Don't let Scooter get near

that thing," I hurriedly said, trying to get off the phone.

When Brian and I were visiting Bear Creek Ranch, I'd made the comment to Bill Beck that will live in infamy with Peggy.

"Heh Billy," I'd said, "If you ever run across a big bear skull will you send it to me?"

When I arrived at the house and found a brown cardboard box on our front steps, a chill ran down my spine. It was thoroughly soaked with blood, even leaving some behind on our freshly painted porch. I couldn't believe the U.S. Mail would deliver such a package. Well, they really lived up to their "Rain or Shine, Sleet or Snow" slogan this time, I mused.

The box was about the size and weight of a case of beer. I pulled it onto the lawn where the blood soaked bottom wouldn't be a problem. When I tore open the top of the box, I fell back with a start. Inside was a bear's head. With ears back and teeth bared, this sickly, deadly, rotten smelling bear's head looked like it was going to lunge out and tear at my throat. The bottom of the box had an inch of blood pooling around it. It was just plain gross. After recovering from my initial shock, I pulled a small wad of paper from the throat of the enormous bear. Blood soaked, it read:

> Dear Wild Willy,
> When you were in Montana, you asked me to get you a bear skull. This one was hit by a car and the park service let me cut its head off with a chainsaw I had in my truck. I mailed it right away so it would still be fresh. I think you'll want to clean it.
> > Your Good Buddy,
> > Billy Beck

That afternoon, Dave and Robin Smith stopped over to borrow a canoe from our garage. Robin, a fragile and squeamish lady who was a very good cook, looked at a big pot, with its contents in a rolling boil, on an electric burner in our garage.

"What's cooking, Bill? It smells kind of different."

"Robin, I'm trying something new, an oriental soup of sorts, kind of like bird's nest soup. It's called bear's head soup." Robin laughed at the silliness of my statement. Suddenly, the bear's head in the boiling liquid popped to the surface of the pot staring right into Robin's startled and ever widening eyes. Dave grabbed her by the arm as her knees buckled. He quickly got her out of the garage, away from the smell, away from the glazed stare of the beheaded behemoth.

"I think I need to sit down," she said faintly to Dave as I approached them.

"Well," I said, rubbing my hands together in glee. "I think Peggy's about done cooking breakfast. How does green eggs and ham sound to you guys this morning?"

A few months later I was off to Sigonella, Sicily, for a six month deployment to spy on Soviet and Libyan submarines in the Mediterranean Ocean. If they detected that we were tracking them, then it became a real high stakes game of cat and mouse. I shared a car and a room with Lieutenant Jay "Bird" Hanson, just as we had shared a room together in Bermuda. Whenever we weren't flying, Bird and I were driving our little Fiat all over Sicily. We would go to pizzerias in Catania at the base of Mt. Etna and go to gelaterias (Italian ice cream parlors) in the spectacular coastal resort town of Taormina. We flew, ate, slept, and worked out. We kept that up for months as the Tigers of Patrol Squadron Eight broke every submarine tracking record in the Mediterranean.

On occasion we flew on special missions called "Red Rockets" below the "line of death" that Mohammar Khaddafi had established off his coastline. It seemed like we were being used as bait—like cheese in a mousetrap—just hoping Khaddafi would order his fighters out to attack us so that our F-14s from a nearby aircraft carrier could shoot them down.

We also supported operations off the coast of Lebanon and

watched from the air as the giant 16 inch guns from the Battleship *New Jersey* shelled Lebanon. It was an awesome sight and my longest flight, 13.8 hours from takeoff to landing. I was glad I was not on the receiving end of those monstrous shells and felt a tinge of pain for those that were. A bullet with a 16 inch diameter is a monstrous thing to be filling the skies and it tends to get people's attention—tends to bring them to the negotiating table, so to speak.

While in Sigonella, Sicily, I received orders to fly to Sardinia to be an observer for a week on a nuclear attack submarine, the USS *Whale*. What an amazing ride! The skipper, Commander Welsh, was a terrific host and gave me complete freedom to wander around. The sub was underway during her break-in period called "Sea Trials" so they maneuvered, deep dived and steamed to the *Whale's* very limits.

One evening at about two in the morning, I was alone in the officers' galley watching the German movie *DAS BOOT (The Boat)* about a tour of duty on a Nazi U-boat during WWII. As the submarine in the movie was attacked with depth charges, I was suddenly thrown from my chair as the *Whale* nosed over to do a deep test dive to greater than one thousand feet below the surface of the Mediterranean. As I got up, scratching my head and still studying the video mayhem on board the sinking U-boat, my eyes scanned the depth gauge and the angle of bank indicators on the wardroom's bulkhead. I smelled the sweet fragrance of the ionized air almost dripping from the high humidity of super compression. I shuddered as the walls of the real sub, the *Whale*, groaned under the immense pressure as thousands of tons of seawater tried to collapse its fragile shell. Holy smokes, I thought, this has got to be the most convincing and expensive movie theater Sensurround experience that anyone ever had. I could hear it, feel it, smell it, touch it—it was happening to me—as I watched the German sub crew in the movie react to the Captain's orders to deep dive.

The following morning, the Skipper let me experience driving the sub, called "manning the conn," and also had me with him up on top of the sail as we steamed the *Whale* back into Sardinia. Believe me, it takes a special kind of person to endure several months under water with no individual privacy and nothing but work and sleep for months at a stretch.

WHAM!
Goss Slams into Side of Active Volcano

Late one night in Sigonella, we were awakened for an alert launch, which required all twelve crewmen to be airborne within one hour. The Italian Airport traffic controller had previously given us the unusual order to taxi down to the other end of the runway because the wind had shifted directions due to a heavy rainsquall the airport was encountering. The tower signaled our plane with lights on these special flights so that no radio communication between the airplane and the tower could get intercepted. Instantly, after taking off in the opposite direction than usual, our plane entered heavy clouds and turbulence. We executed the standard right turn departure to avoid hitting 11,000-foot Mt. Etna, Europe's largest active volcano.

Suddenly, as the altimeter indicated we were climbing through 4000 feet, something dawned on me. If we normally executed a right turn after take-off to avoid crashing into Mt. Etna, then when we take-off in the opposite direction, shouldn't we turn left to avoid it instead of right as we had automatically done so many times in the past?

"Holy Shit, Scott!" I screamed to the senior pilot, dubbed "Trampster" by his fellow pilots. "We're flying directly into the side of Mt. Etna!!!" I yanked the yoke as hard as I could into as steep a turn as possible relying completely on our flight instruments in the bumpy, vertigo inducing blackness of the storm. "Oh please, please...please, please, please...don't let it be too late!!!" I prayed as we waited the one minute that it took to completely turn the plane 180-degrees away from our previously disastrous heading. The volcano's peak towered 7000 feet above us, hidden somewhere in the dark clouds. I don't know how close we got to impact but it couldn't have been too far away. And since this flight had required that we take off in secret, without putting out any electronic emissions that would have helped the Italian air traffic controllers track us—or warn us—we had been literally and figuratively flying in the dark.

We landed thirteen hours later. Trampster and I sat down for a beer and privately commiserated over our terribly close call. The other ten-crew members were clueless to the horrifyingly catastrophic error that we had almost made. It was definitely a case of "familiarity breeds contempt," a common and insidious problem in which all seasoned aviators can relate. In no other field of endeavor is this expression any more meaningful or any deadlier than in aviation—none.

Two days later, to lighten up our somber mood, Trampster and I removed the front seats from our commanding officer's car and installed two toilet seats in their place. We thought it was a good practical joke until Skipper Figueras caught us. He then ordered us to reinstall his driver side car seat, yet insisted we leave the passenger side toilet seat in place. For the rest of the week, he proudly drove his official vehicle around the Navy base with his executive officer, Commander Andy Gabriel, sitting next to him perched high up on that toilet seat. It did a lot for morale. Well, maybe not the Executive Officer's, but the junior officers loved it.

WHAM!
Goss Plane Hit by Titan Missiles

A few months later, after completing our deployment in Sicily, I was sent as the senior pilot with my crew down to Barbados for a special operation called "SMILS." It stood for "Sonobuoy Missile Impact Location System." From Barbados we flew a thousand miles out into a remote part of the South Atlantic carrying a special group of scientists with expensive photographic and listening equipment, nuclear clocks, and stuff that I'm still clueless about. Arriving at sunset, one of the scientists helped guide me to an exact position 8000 feet over the South Atlantic on an exact heading. Looking at his precision timepiece, he stated "5, 4, 3, 2, 1, now look out front." As I searched the heavens, a host of white specks lined across my windshield. They grew brighter and brighter until they all looked like a noon sun. Then, like a demonic tiger scratching claws of fire down the center of the P-3 Orion's windshield, a multitude of nuclear warheads poured from the sky, like twelve shooting stars, just a few miles from my plane. "Holy Shit," my flight engineer exclaimed as he snapped pictures. It was the most unbelievable sight I hope to never see again—a possible early look at a future Armageddon. The missiles had been part of a practice launch from a submerged U.S. submarine, a "Boomer," minutes earlier and thousands of miles away. The launch command had probably been given from the White House, with, I would hope, a quick courtesy call to the Kremlin first. I was able to capture all of it on film, the orbital reentry of twelve Trident II missile warheads glowing, nearly burning up, as they hit the friction of the Earth's atmosphere at well over ten times the speed of sound. The splashes they made into the ocean below us must have been hundreds of feet high.

Silently, we turned back to Barbados, as the scientists evaluated the impact sounds of the test MIRVs (multiple independently targeted re-entry vehicles) to determine the accuracy of our Trident II missile delivery system. Testing perfectly, all the "vehicles" were bulls-eyes. Leave it to some highly paid bureaucrat to come up with the innocuous sounding term "vehicle" to describe our country's most devastating weapon of mass destruction, a nuclear warhead.

Test launch or not, that experience was an incredibly sobering sight. Ever since that night, seeing shooting stars heading my way on dark nights still causes me to ponder as my eyes follow them in their fall to the earth. It was then that I realized that the world as we know it could be ended by a simple command from a world leader—"Launch 'Em."

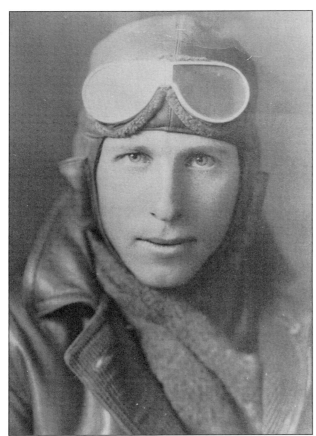

Charles L. Dacey (1894–1992) Army Signal Corps Aviator. Incredibly talented—and funny—he ended his flying career in 1918 because "Billy, there just wasn't any future in it." He came to this conclusion after his best friend was killed in a JN-4 "Jenny" plane crash. My mentor, "Pop," lived to be 97. Maybe Pop was right, at least in regards to the life expectancy of pilots at that time.

World War I's most famous airplane, the JN-4 "Jenny." This is the plane Pop flew.

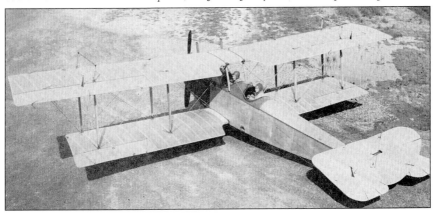

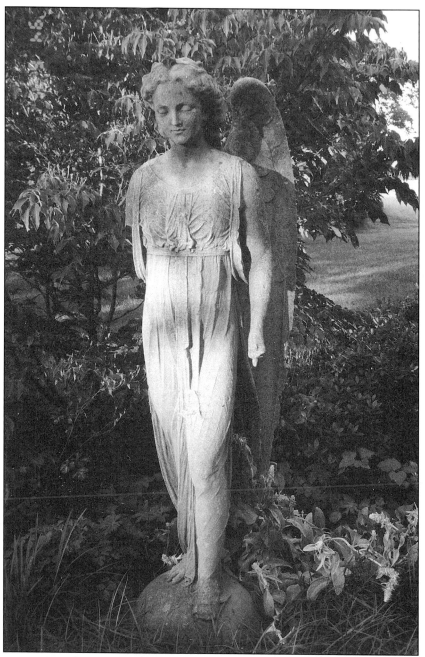

My grandfather carved this 8-foot angel as a headstone for his young daughter who died of pneumonia. My father remembers watching his father work on the giant slab of stone whenever he had free time, month after month, year after year, in their tiny backyard in Newark, New Jersey.

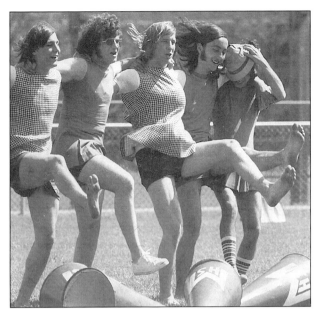

After acquiring the cheerleader uniforms, my buddies and I gave the cheerleaders an impromptu lesson on how to conduct cheers.

Cubie after a successful hunt with four dead Gabers ready to be stuffed and mounted.

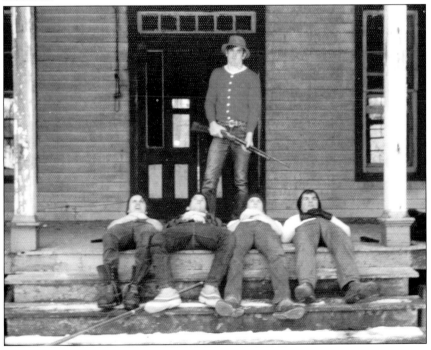

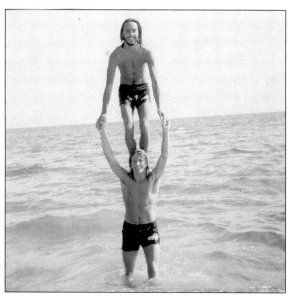

Jungle James and I taking a break from Millburn
High School in the surf at the Jersey shore.

Peggy after some skin diving lessons in "The Lake."

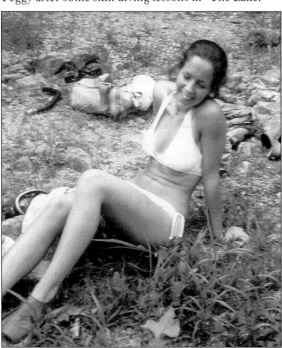

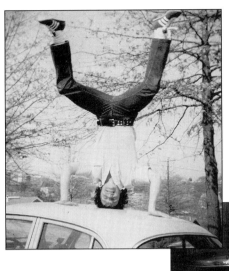

Rat on top of Festus, the Volvo Amazon I bought for $80 and drove one hundred thousand miles.

Gureenie and Cubie belt out a number for Maid Marian.

The men and then some. Cubie's bachelor party.

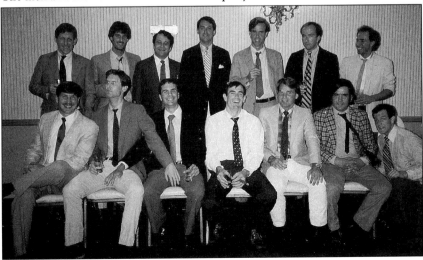

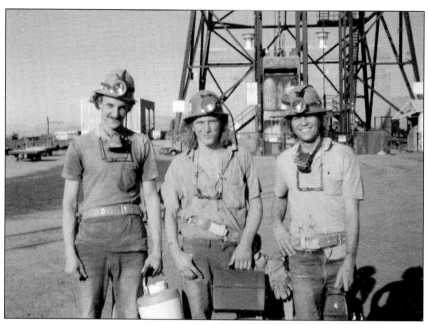

Larry Rayko, Dave Pash and I at the top of the copper mine where I almost got crushed. Behind us is the elevator shaft that dropped thousands of feet per minute.

Rat, Jungle James and I on one of our sick adventures. This time we climbed across the half fallen down train tressel behind us, then had to swim across the rapids to get back.

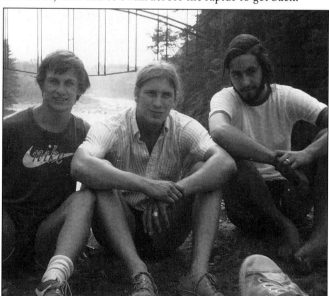

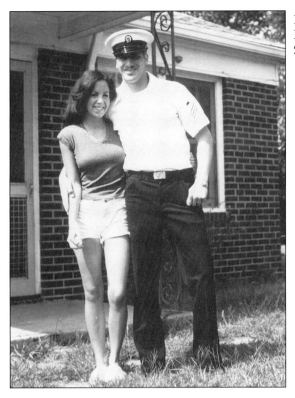

Peggy and I, a U.S. Navy Mineman, in Charleston, South Carolina.

Leaning against a truck full of 2,000 lb. mines full of high explosives. A short time later these huge bombs fell off the back of the truck when it blew a tire in a turn.

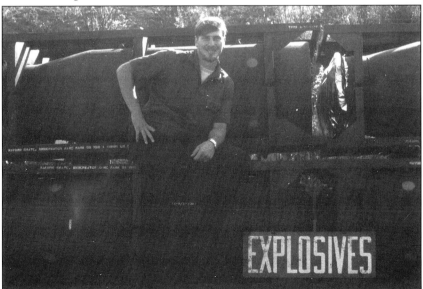

Winning the base boxing smoker by a knockout. My poor opponent, lying on his side, had to be carried out of the ring.

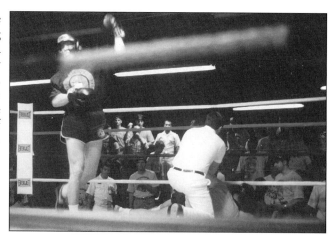

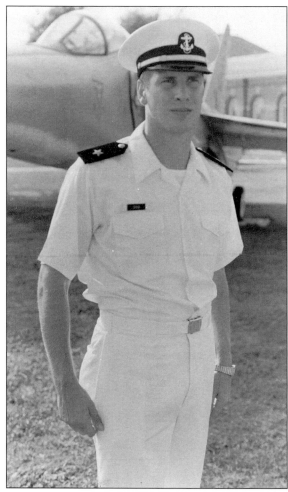

Naval Aviation Officer Candidate William A. Goss at Naval Air Station, Pensacola, Florida.

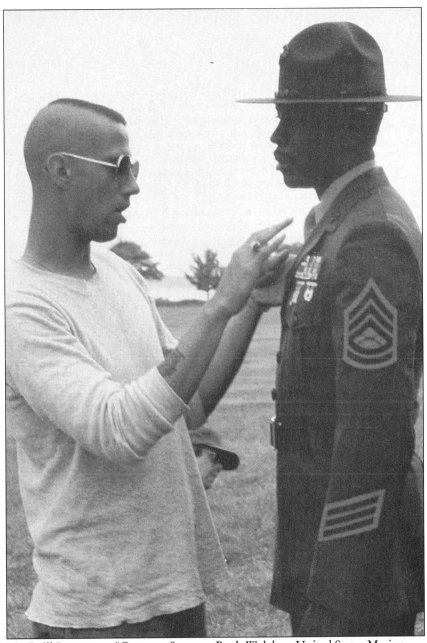

My Drill Instructor, "Gunnery Sergeant Buck Welcher, United States Marine Corps, Sir," giving advice to Lou Gossett, Jr. on the set of *An Officer and a Gentleman*, where Buck spent two months leave serving as technical director. Lou Gossett won an Academy Award for Best Supporting Actor.

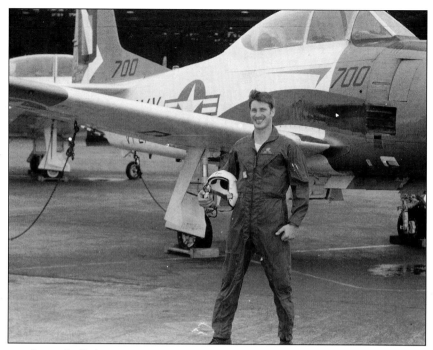

My first solo flight.

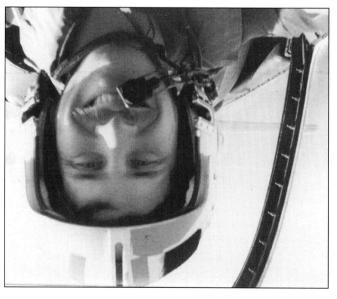

Flying
upside
down in
the T-28
Trojan.

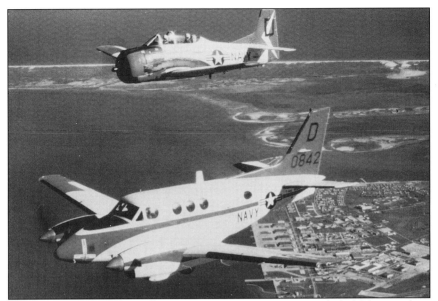

Two planes I spent a lot of time training in over Corpus Christi, Texas—the T-28 Trojan and the T-44 Pegasus.

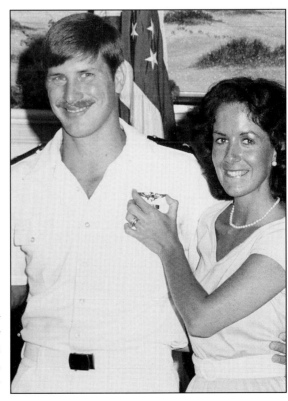

Peggy pinning on my brand new Navy Wings of Gold in Corpus Christi, Texas.

Here is a picture of me flying the P-3 Orion down the Amazon River of Brazil. It was taken the moment we crossed the equator.

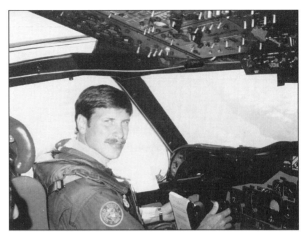

P-3 Orion loaded with Harpoon anti-ship missiles. Its bomb bay doors are open.

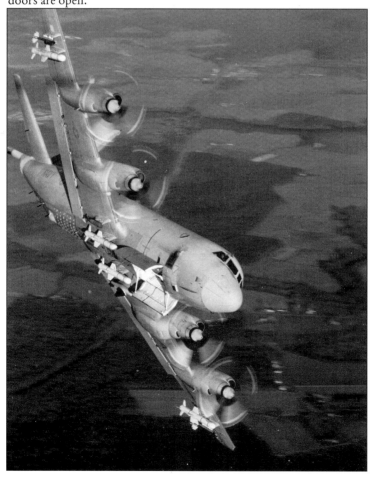

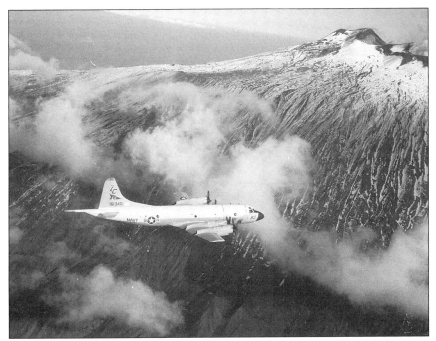

A Patrol Squadron Eight P-3 Orion flying by 11,000 foot Mt. Etna, Europe's largest active volcano. We almost flew into the side of it during bad weather at night.

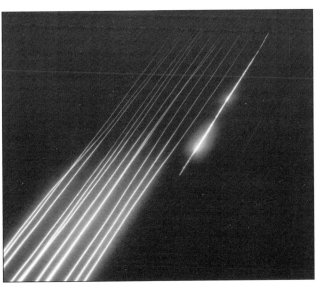

This is what it might look like in the skies moments before the end of the world. This photo, of 12 nuclear warheads reentering the atmosphere at ten times the speed of sound, was taken from the cockpit of the plane I was flying in the center of the South Atlantic.

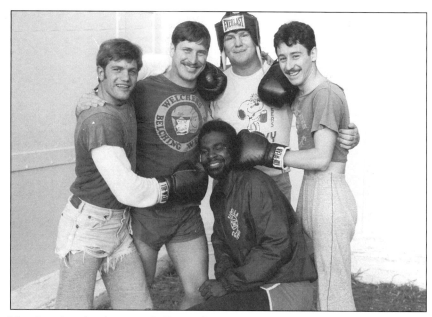

My victorious boxing team in Bermuda.

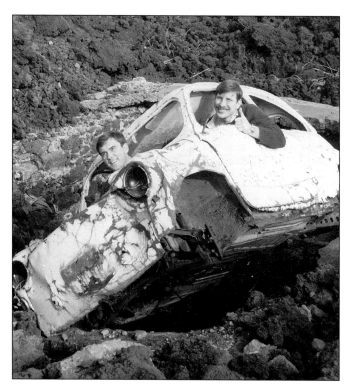

Bird and I in an old Fiat stuck in the lava flows of Mt. Etna, Sicily.

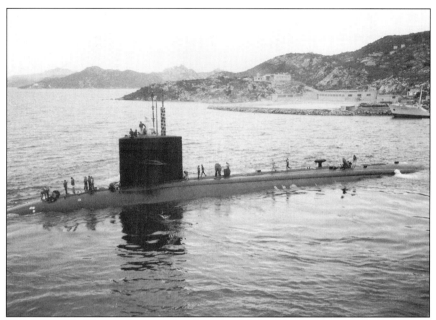

USS *WHALE*—The nuclear attack submarine I joined in Sardinia and rode for a week of sea trials in the Mediterranean.

Peggy, Scooter and I with the bear skull that I had just completed cleaning the meat off of by boiling it in hot water for hours out in our garage.

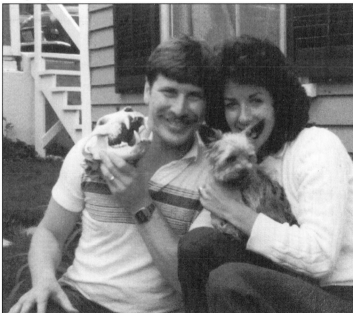

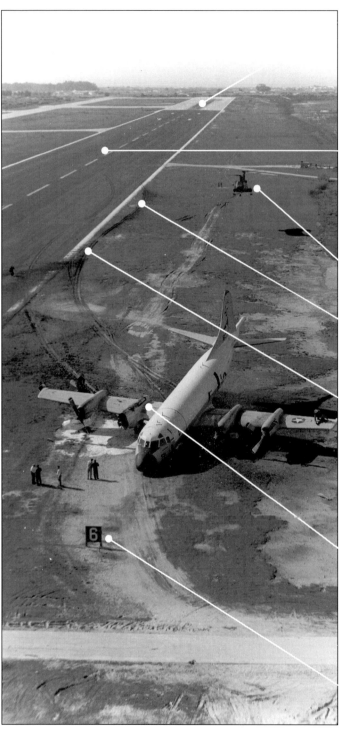

Pilot at the controls makes a simulated 3-engine landing, perfect touch-down on center-line at 145 mph.

At 7000 ft. of runway remaining, the aircraft snaps off runway (note skid marks) within 2 seconds.

Airborne helicopter taking photos.

In 2 seconds I snapped aircraft back towards the runway.

Unbeknownst to anyone but himself, the flight engineer shut down the #1 engine and the airplane uncontrollably snapped violently to the left.

When #3 propeller hit the dirt it tore #3 engine off the wing and snapped the 100,000 lb. airplane 90° to the right.

This sign indicates 6000 ft. of runway remaining.

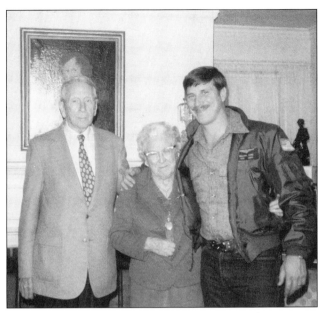

My grandparents, Charles Dacey, an Army Signal Corps pilot in 1918, my grandmother Francis T. Dacey and I.

An informal Goss family reunion on the steps of my sister Peggy and my brother-in-law Howard's home.

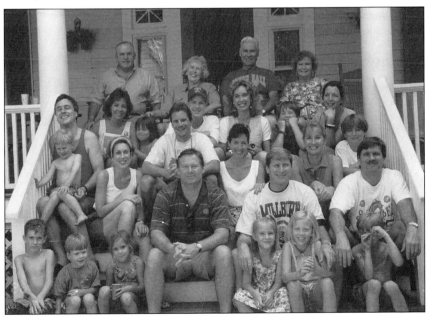

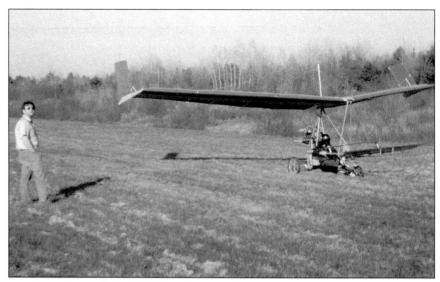

I'm flying the Pterodactyl, an ultralight airplane I flew in Maine and in Texas.

Getting ready for a flight in the AH-1 Cobra gunship helicopter.

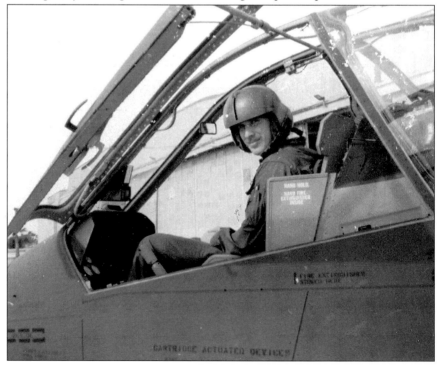

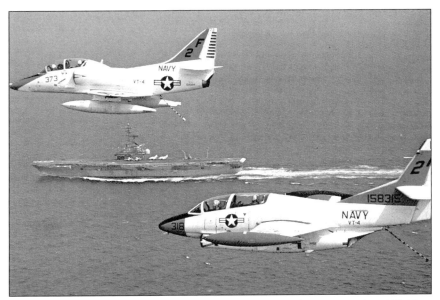

The TA-4 Skyhawk and the T-2 Buckeye with the aircraft carrier USS LEXING-TON in the background. I landed on "Lady Lex" in both of these aircraft.

Flying close formation in the TA-4 Skyhawk.

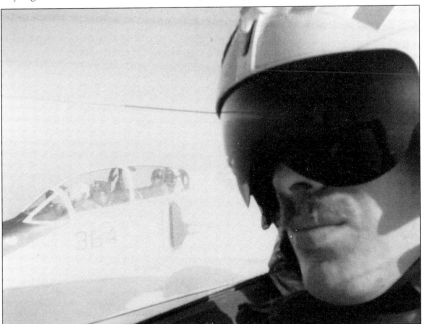

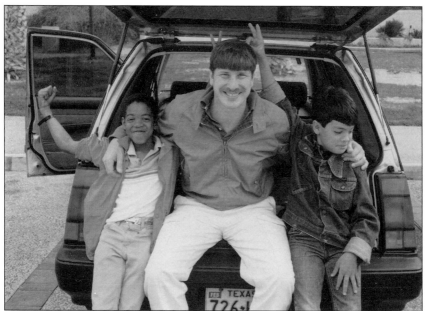

Anthony, my "Little Brother" Andrew Hill and I sitting on the back of the Honda Civic that took Peggy and I for quite a spin a few nights later. As part of the Big Brother Program, Andrew and I shared hobbies and played a variety of sports over the course of three years.

Brian and Christie's first Christmas. We sent this out as a "Season's Greeting" card. Note, along with Scooter, I have a red ratsnake around my neck.

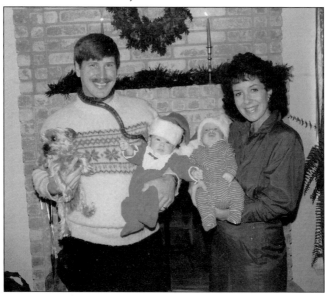

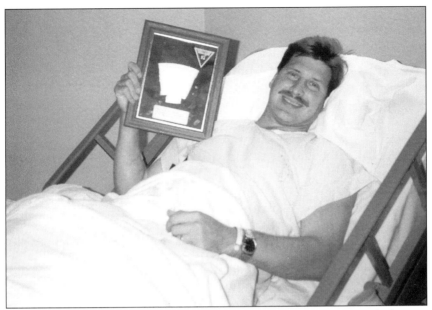

In the hospital after being struck by the out-of-control Ford Fairlane. The letter of commendation read, "To Commander Roadkill Goss—For Being in the Conspicuous Line of a Car."

With close friend USMC Captain Bruce Hilgartner of Squadron VFA-106, after we broke the sound barrier off the coast of Jacksonville.

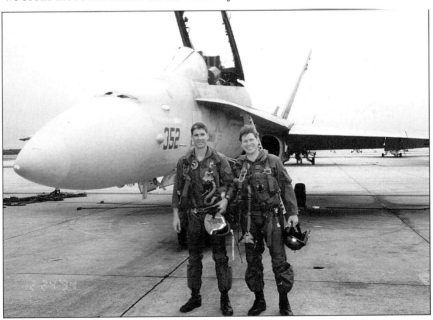

The healing
process
begins after
11 hours of
surgery.

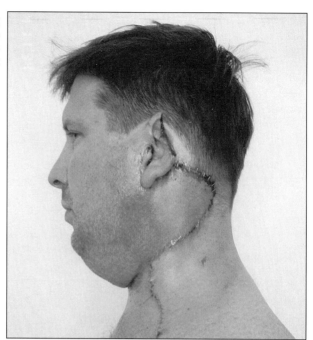

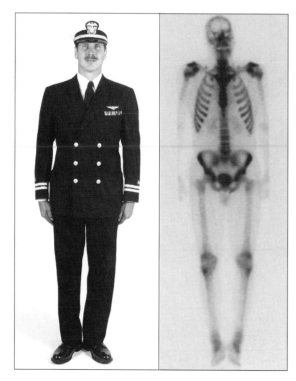

Standing tall next to
my full body bone
scan. I have them to
determine if the
malignancy is spread-
ing to my bones. They
would light up white if
the cancer is spreading.

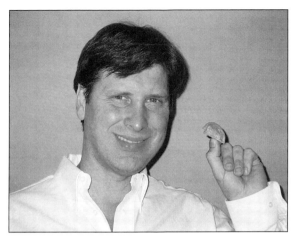

My fake ear that I used Duco cement to hold in place. The nice ladies in the cosmetics department at Dillard's covered it with makeup to try to make it look real.

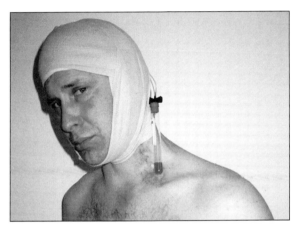

Ear reconstruction surgery post-op. Some of my top right rib was removed and placed under my skin on the side of my head. Son Brian told me "Daddy, don't go outside—you'll be pecked to death by humming-birds!"

My left groin—just one of the places where the meat for my new left ear came from.

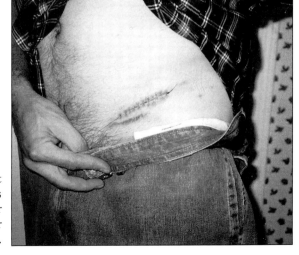

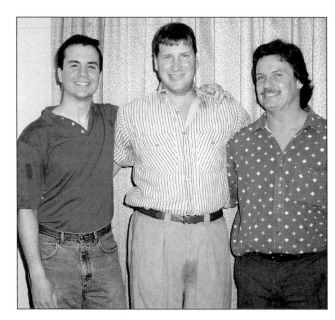

A night out on the town soon after surgery with Gureenie (aka ear, nose and throat surgeon and childhood buddy, Dr. Carl Guarino), me and, oh yeah, Dr. Rat. Check out the wet spot on my crotch. It is actually saliva that dripped down off my chin from a hole that would not heal behind what remained of my left ear.

Whitewater rafting down the Colorado River with the team from Panavision International. (clockwise L-R) Bill Scott, Freebs, Grazzoo, Boobus, Bob Sherman, David Scott, and I.

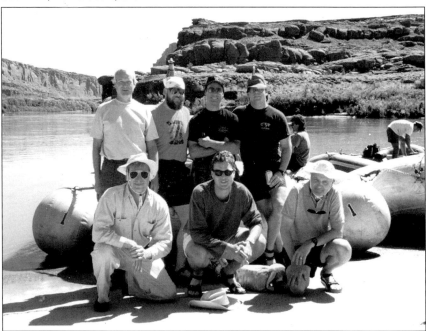

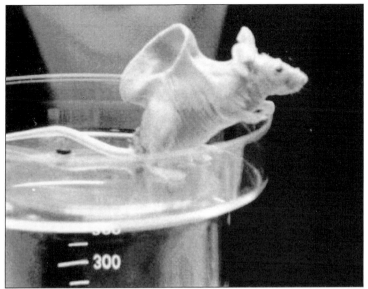

A new patent-pending biogenetically engineered nude mouse with a human ear growing out of its back. Unfortunately, this is a right-eared mouse, but I'm sure that a left-eared one is on the drawing board. (Courtesy of AP/Wide World photos)

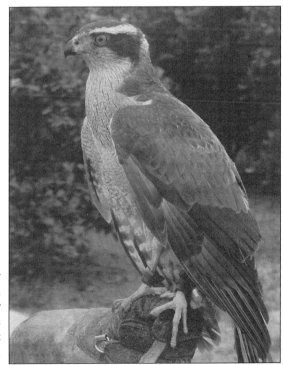

A Goshawk on my hand is worth two in the bush. Pound for pound, this is nature's most powerful predator.

Myself and Rudy Ruettiger, a close friend and the Notre Dame football inspiration behind TriStar's blockbuster movie, *RUDY*.

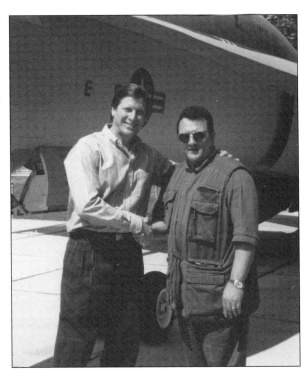

Hummer, the hummingbird that lived in our guest bedroom for a few weeks, on my thumb.

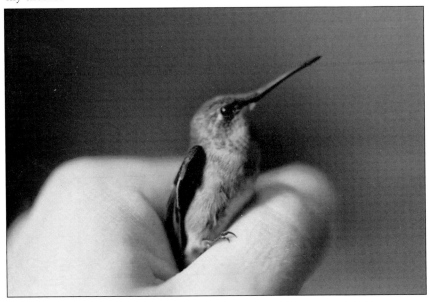

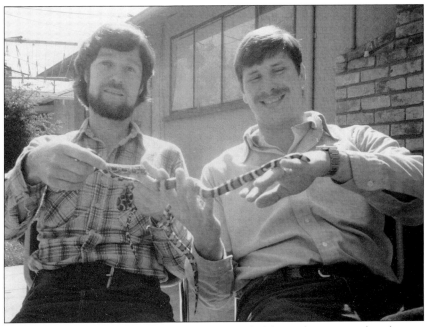

Snakeman and I with either a gorgeous mountain kingsnake or a coral snake.

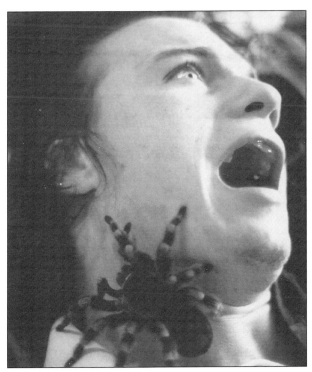

Rat and his pet
tarantula, Igor.

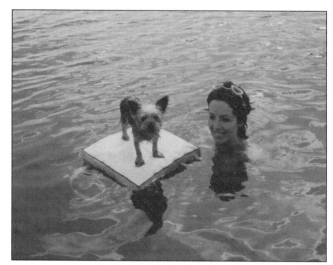

Peggy, with Scooter adrift on a lifeseat, swimming behind our house on Padre Island, Texas.

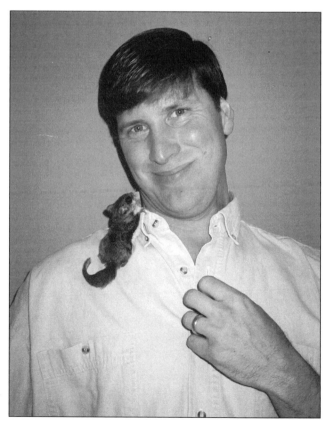

Rocky J. Flying Squirrel and Billwinkle.

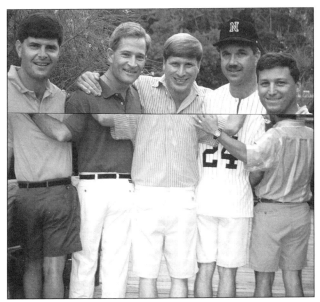

The BOBS—Big Old Butts—A club for back assward Naval Officers.

My brothers and sisters in back of brother Bob's home in Oldwick, New Jersey. (L-R) Larry, me, Bob, Mimi, Peggy and Jackie.

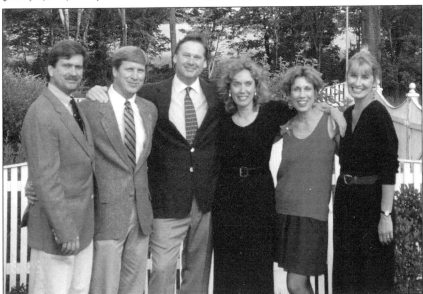

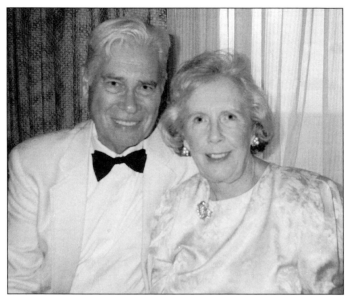

My parents, Eugene and Barbara Goss, on their 45th wedding anniversary.

Our Christmas photo seven months after my eleven-hour radical neck dissection surgery for malignant melanoma.

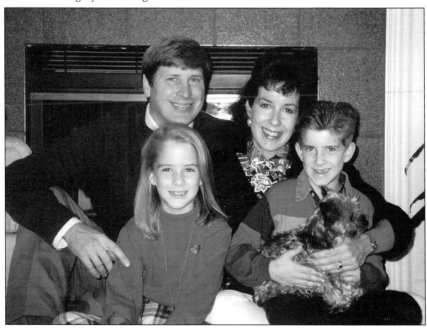

Approach Magazine carried the following article I wrote about an experience I had as Patrol Plane Commander a short time later. It will give you a taste of military aviation lingo. We were dropping inert 2000-pound mines off the coast of Charleston and I was flying the lead P-3C. The sun was rising right in my face and it was blinding. The sky was filled with seagulls.

THOSE AREN'T SEAGULLS—
THEY'RE WART HOGS!
By Lt. Bill Goss, U.S. Navy

Three P-3C Orions were making their final VFR (Visual Flight Rules) run, at a mining range off the coast of South Carolina. It had been reserved exclusively for this squadron all afternoon. The three previous computer on-line runs had been uneventful, with the normal abundance of coastal bird activity. The last run of the day was to be a slightly more difficult simulated off-line drop. The winter afternoon sun had started to sit lower on the horizon and this next off-line run was directly into it. Occasional seagulls had been successfully avoided throughout the previous runs. At push time the lead P-3C descended to 300 feet, accelerated to 300 knots and commenced flight toward the initial point (IP) directly into the glare of the sun. The patrol plane commander (PPC) spotted two seagulls in the distance. They appeared a few hundred feet above them in their flight path. They would easily fly below and between them. The co-pilot and the flight engineer acknowledged the birdcall and concurred that the birds would be "no factor."

Moments later, now at the start of the mine line and in the direct glare of the sun, the flight station again checked the position of the two seagulls. Again, "no factor," they wouldn't be flying any nearer to them than any other birds they had seen today at 300 feet and 300 knots. Seconds later, the birds appeared to grow shockingly in size and had really mastered picture perfect spread wing formation flight. As these particular "seagulls" instantly filled the field of view from the cockpit it dawned on the entire flight station. . . . "Those aren't seagulls. . .they're A-10s!"

The two camouflage-painted Air Force A-10 "wart hog" attack jets were flying directly up the P-3s reserved practice mine line. The lead P-3 was now head-on but still apparently passing below and splitting the difference between the A-10s with less than one-mile distance at a closing speed of approximately 600 knots. The PPC elected to maintain heading. Diversive action to starboard or port would have put him into either the water below or head-on into the A-10 wart hog on each side of him. They just missed having a mid-air collision.

LESSON LEARNED: A-10 wart hogs really do look like seagulls when approached head-on. This illusion fooled two pilots and a Flight Engineer for an unsafe period of time (approximately 20 seconds). A-10s also like to fly very low along the coast just like seagulls. The only way to tell the difference head-on is that the green spread wing A-10 fills up your windscreen about a thousand times faster. Direct sun in your eyes doesn't help. Try to avoid flying the mining profile directly into the sun. Personally call military air commands in the vicinity of mining ranges and inform them that multiple P-3s will be flying a high speed/low altitude VFR profile along a specific track in reserved airspace. Also, the spacing you give birds is not the spacing to give airplanes. Near midairs are not filed on close approaches with seagulls. If there is any doubt as to the identity of an approaching UFO, give it plenty of space.

Finally, VFR is VFR, so keep your head out of the cockpit; avoid flying into the sun; and stay out of the way of anything that looks like seagulls (no matter how good a bird dodger you might think you are), because your flock of seagulls might turn into a flight of wart hogs before you can blink an eye.

After those two A-10 wart hogs tried to make an Air Force sandwich out of us off the coast of Charleston, things calmed down for a few months while our squadron, the VP-8 Tigers, prepared for another deployment—this one being to Rota, Spain.

"Far better it is to dare mighty things,
to win glorious triumphs,
even though checkered with failure,
than to take ranks with those poor spirits
who neither enjoy much nor suffer much,
because they live in the gray twilight
that knows not victory or defeat."
—Teddy Roosevelt

CHAPTER SIX

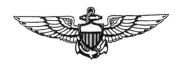

WHAM!
GOSS "BENDS THE METAL"

"A person's character is not made in a crisis,
it is only exhibited then."
—Author Unknown

A n old aviation expression goes something like this: "There are those that have bent metal and there are those that will." This little rose of wisdom leaves no possibility that a pilot will never be involved in an aircraft mishap. I found this thought quite remarkable since I figured good pilots would not, could not, be involved in a crash. And I was a good pilot.

A few days after arriving in Rota, Spain, my copilot and I and our brand new third pilot were scheduled for a few hours of landing practice, known as "touch and goes" by Navy pilots. It was on this day when I "bent the metal" and learned the true wisdom of that old aviation expression. The crash and the ensuing investigation is fully described in an article I wrote which was honored with the "Outstanding Article of the Year" award after it was published in *Approach* magazine. Here is a condensed version of that article:

PILOT IN COMMAND VS.
PILOT AT THE CONTROLS
By Lt. Bill Goss, U.S. Navy

I was scheduled for a few hours of touch-and-go

landings and take-offs with a copilot who rarely agreed with anything I said. We had just had a heated disagreement about the previous day's post-maintenance check flight, but I'd hoped that this flight in the P-3C Orion would somehow improve our relationship because the landings and takeoffs demand clear communications and understanding among the crew.

I was in the right seat, and the copilot was in the left seat. Our plan was to give the copilot eight touch-and-goes with the last being a full stop to drop him off. We had been lulled by the beautiful weather, the smooth touch-and-goes and our own efforts at resolving our internal conflicts with one another. It was less than an ideal posture for simulating an emergency.

Both of us considered a simulated three-engine landing a relatively easy thing to do. We had not learned the subtle things that an instructor pilot (IP) might do during this maneuver to prevent an overly dramatic reduction in controllability, something that happens during simulated engine out work at air speeds below VMC ground (velocity of minimum control on the ground) of 115 mph. Rolling final, with the #4 engine set near flight idle to simulate that the engine was not operating, the aircraft was set up nicely on the extended runway centerline and with proper airspeeds.

Touchdown was ideal, at about 145 mph and on centerline. I commended the copilot on his touchdown and cautioned him to take it easy going into reverse, especially since we had a long way to roll out before turning off the runway to drop him off. After rolling out at least 2,000 feet, the copilot lifted all four power levels up over the throttle ramp. He pulled power levers #1, #2 and #3 toward maximum reverse. #4 power lever was not pulled back far enough to get a beta light, indicating that thrust would still be positive rather than negative on that engine.

Unfortunately, this fact was not announced as required by the flight engineer nor recognized by any of the pilots. The aircraft had slowed to below VMC ground, meaning that the rudder was about to lose all effectiveness in maintaining centerline control.

As the P-3C yawed slightly left of centerline, the copilot fed in the last remaining inch of right rudder. This action momentarily reestablished centerline, but had unfortunately wasted our last remaining bit of rudder authority. The right rudder was now tight against the floorboard. A fraction of a second later the aircraft snapped violently to the left of the runway centerline.

As the right seat pilot and pilot in command (PIC), I now stated loudly that I wanted to be pilot at the controls as well. In less than two seconds, our left main mount had gone four feet off the runway and in the dirt at a speed of 100 mph. What I would have given for a little more concrete on the left side of the runway!

After a momentary struggle on the controls with the copilot, who thought it was his responsibility to get us out of this mess, I set maximum power on engines #1 and #2 and made a corrective swerve back to the right toward runway centerline. I was confident that I had saved the day—and the airplane.

Suddenly the aircraft snapped left more violently than before. It departed the left side of the runway, twisting off the landing gear and causing the #3 propeller to touch the ground. That instantly tore the entire 4600-shaft horsepower engine propeller assembly off the aircraft. I remember seeing it out of the corner of my eye as it flew by over the right wing.

It could not have taken more than eight seconds to go from being perfectly on the runway centerline—to having the left main mount four feet off the side of the runway—to having reestablished control and having moved back toward the runway—to having finally snapped to the left and ultimately crashed. Pulling the Emergency Engine Shutdown handles and evacuating the badly damaged aircraft probably took another 15 seconds. Luckily, no one was hurt.

What caused the final disastrous snap to the left? I found out two days later—the flight engineer had reached up and shut down the #1 engine on which I had max power set in an effort to move back to the right toward centerline. The resulting drag, with a windmilling propeller condition on the left side and positive thrust on the right side, now made the crash to the left impossible to prevent.

Immediately after the mishap, crewmembers

were separated and prevented from talking to one another. The accident investigation, JAG investigation, medical inquiries, Field Naval Aviation Evaluation Board (FNAEB) and aircraft repair work were time-consuming. The grand finale of the three-month ordeal was the FNAEB making me realize the simple point that, no matter what other crew members may do to cause an aircraft mishap, it is not their responsibility. The responsibility for the safe completion of a flight or for a mishap rests solely with the man who signs the "A" sheet: the Pilot In Command (PIC). Although that was a bitter pill to swallow, it proved to be a valuable lesson.

Pilots, don't assume the crew knows what you are thinking and you know what they are thinking. Communicate. If efforts to communicate with certain crewmembers fail, recommend a crew change before a communication breakdown causes an accident. Ask yourself: "What if?" The more possible scenarios you have reviewed as a crew, the less surprised you will be when a "what if" becomes a "what now?"

Make sure all pilots on board know that when the PIC says, "I've got the airplane," controls need to be passed immediately. Intentionally delaying the passing of aircraft control to the PIC in situations where split seconds may count is not only unsafe but also insubordinate. On the other hand, the PIC should realize that despite all the training, co-pilots are human.

Being involved in an aircraft mishap as the Pilot In Command is one of the most miserable experiences that one can go through. Do whatever you have to do to avoid placing the aircraft and crew in a potential mishap situation. However, if you end up in a mishap and survive, take you licks, learn as much as possible, get on with your life and don't give up flying. It will not only become fun again but will probably become a lot safer for you as well. You cannot make your accident "un-happen." To quote my old Executive Officer's favorite expression, "You can only play with the hand that's dealt you."

The Accident Board concluded that once I had maneuvered the airplane back towards the centerline of the runway all the Flight Engineer had to do was just sit there and enjoy the ride. I would have brought the airplane to a stop on the runway with little or no damage to it. Instead he decided to try something new and unique by instantly shutting down the one engine that I was relying on most to keep us on the runway.

Yet, I was stuck in the untenable situation of having to assume complete responsibility and accountability for the inexplicable actions of others—even though I felt I had no control over their completely unexpected responses. My sense of anger, frustration and denial almost overwhelmed me.

I came to realize that being a Pilot In Command is often like being a parent—even though you did your best raising your children, when they screw up someone still has to step in and assume responsibility for what went wrong. And of course my Commanding Officer had to feel the same way about me. It was a bitter but important pill for a brand new lieutenant to swallow. As you can imagine, I never again felt really comfortable with Flight Engineers sitting behind me, out of view, within arm's reach of those damn engine shutdown switches. But who would after an experience like that?

Peggy learned of this incident minutes after it happened with the phone call, "Peggy, there's been a mishap..." and she heard about it on ABC News as well. She flew to Spain to be with me a few days later.

The initial cost estimate using new replacement parts for all damages was set at $3.5 million and I expected every penny of it to come out of my hide. I felt so ashamed and such remorse at having played a part in the trashing of the Skipper's new plane that I just wanted to crawl under a rock and die. I had never known before that shame was such a powerful emotion. It can make you hurt all over like you have a debilitating illness. I was devastated by having to accept the blame for an accident that I felt should not have happened. It was the closest I have ever come to wanting to die.

If you saw the movie *Top Gun*, you saw the board of inquiry and hellacious experience that Tom Cruise's character went through on the silver screen. Imagine going through all that in real life. Thankfully nobody was hurt and, after a six-month repair job, the airplane ultimately flew again. It was with this mishap in my last two months with the Tigers of Patrol Squadron Eight, that I concluded what had been, until this event, a very successful first pilot tour. It was the worst possible way to end things. A parting shot from a philosophical squadronmate of mine said it all, "So long, Bill—when all else fails, fame can be assured by spectacular error."

With this monkey on my back, Peggy and I loaded the old black Volvo Amazon, left Maine, and headed for Corpus Christi, Texas, where the Navy still wanted me to be a flight instructor. I felt I would have to prove myself all over again. I had to be the best. Pilots' egos are like that, and sometimes it's not the healthiest of things, at least where the families are concerned.

At first, it was difficult going through the T-44 aircraft instructor syllabus so soon after my challenging learning experience in Rota, Spain, but somehow I made it through. In fact, I became an instructor in two new programs, the "C2/E2" syllabus for aircraft carrier designated students and also in the T-44 "Formation Flight" syllabus. I ended up having to learn how to teach formation flying from another senior lieutenant with whom I had a lot of personal run-ins. Plus after the Rota, Spain incident, I was uncomfortable with the concept of banging up another plane. As much as I loved to fly, I have to admit I was never a "natural." Learning new maneuvers never came easily to me. What I didn't have in natural ability, I always figured I could make up for with practice, perseverance and hard work. And when that didn't do it—more hard work.

Consequently, it took me some additional time to get the hang of the "rendezvous," one of the more dangerous aspects of formation flying. Thanks to my Commanding Officer's encouragement and guidance, I became a pretty good formation instructor rather than a washout.

In time, I began to excel as an instructor pilot and was honored with the squadron's "Instructor of the Quarter" award, the Navy League's "Officer of the Year" award, and also a Navy Achievement Medal. The flying was fantastic, as students and I flew all over the United States on training flights that were terrific learning experiences for both the "studs" (as the student pilots were known) and myself. Whenever we flew over the Grand Canyon, I would get radar clearance down to as low as we could legally go. It gave the stud a chance to relax and enjoy the beauty and spectacle of flight over one of God's most beautiful and spectacular creations. I instructed male and female students from the United States Marines, the Coast Guard and the Navy. I also instructed studs from the foreign militaries of Italy, Norway and even Jersey City—which was where Franco Lo Piccollo, one of my favorite studs, was from. An American guy more Italian than the eight students sent over from Italy.

Corpus Christi Naval Air Station had some of the busiest airspace in the world. Keeping our heads on a swivel and our eyes constantly scanning between instrument panels and the congested airspace outside the cockpit was an essential part of flight instructing. A good "scan" helped to prevent a deadly collision with radio towers, mountains, other flying aircraft, and large birds. Luck also helped.

During that tour, I filed several near mid-air collision reports against other aircraft and many bird strike reports including one with a giant turkey vulture that we struck as it glided across the runway moments before my airplane touched down. If we hit that bird at a higher speed it would have spelled disaster for my student and me. Vultures sometimes strike an aircraft's windshield so hard that it shatters, blasting glass and ten pounds of bird at hundreds of miles per hour into the face of the totally astounded pilot. Astounded that is, if the pilot is not killed.

Problems relating to bird strikes happen with regularity to military pilots. It was supposedly a strike from a small bird that brought down a $300 million B-1 bomber. I've heard of bat strikes and I've even heard of a rattlesnake strike. Evidently a hawk dropped one onto the windshield of an airplane flying below it. A fellow instructor pilot I worked with once struck a full-grown bull while landing at a remote field one dark night. It destroyed the plane, instantly killed the bull, and earned the pilot the dubious nickname "Butcher," which, being a vegetarian, he despised.

While in Texas, my jet instructor buddies helped get me the opportunity to log stick time and carrier landings with them on the aircraft carrier USS Lexington. I did this flying the T-2 Buckeye and TA-4 Skyhawk jets. From the air, Lady Lex looked like a postage stamp bobbing on the surface of the ocean. Moments later, we were on top of her at 600 feet, in a near vertical, 5 G turn to reduce airspeed. We'd call "the ball" (the meatball was a green light mounted on the deck of the ship that visually allows the pilot at the controls to position the aircraft on a safe glidepath) as we intercepted the proper glideslope while at the same time "rolling into the groove." In a rapid descent for twenty seconds, we'd be in a controlled crash landing onto Lady Lex's deck. Jerked violently to a stop by one of four arresting cables stretched across the deck, we'd decelerate from 150 to 0 mph in less than a second.

After a minute or two of following taxiing instructions from an eighteen year old sailor who held our lives in his hands, we'd get hooked up to the catapult for a 0 to 185 mph two second catshot. The hydraulic catapult of the old Lexington kicked like a mule when compared to the slightly softer, steam catapults of the more technologically advanced nuclear aircraft carrier. A proper night landing (called an "OK" pass if it's perfect) required touching down on a bobbing, weaving, vertigo inducing forty foot long patch, stuck in the middle of a bunch of parked planes way out somewhere in the middle of the friggin' ocean with almost no visual references. Mixing the difficulty of a normal carrier landing with a combination of rain, snow, turbulence, hail, engine malfunctions, low fuel and no place else to land can create a high degree of anxiety. It's often more stressful than flying actual combat missions into enemy gunfire. Besides flying the space shuttle, "cats and traps" has got to be an aviator's top thrill ride. Pulling 5 G's feels like one thousand pounds of pressure because—technically speaking—it is. Tactical carrier aviators who do this kind of flying day in and day out are the most competitive and talented aviators in the world. They thrive on adversity. Getting the opportunity to land and takeoff from an aircraft carrier was an incredible experience— one that a simulator could never effectively duplicate. Having fellow flight instructors cross-train me in jets—and even in helicopters like the Army's AH-1 Cobra, the Navy's UH-1 Uhuey and the Coast Guard's HH-65 Dauphine—was one of the best parts about being a Navy pilot. Each and every aircraft provided its own unique and wild ride.

After a year in the squadron, I was assigned duties as the T-44 Model Manager. In this job, I ensured that all engineering and flight procedures were sound for the Navy's T-44 Pegasus aircraft. I also conducted the flight testing of the military instructor pilots designated to teach in this category of plane. It was a great job for a lieutenant. Jim Keen, a U.S. Navy test pilot, was typical of most of the commanding officers I served. He was warm, intelligent and born to excel under almost any circumstance. His wife Susan was just as dynamic as he. Most of the aviators I knew who had the drive to make it to the more senior command positions were extraordinarily talented individuals and gifted leaders. Being that kind of guy, Jim refused to sit back and watch any of his junior officers falter. To sum it up, he cared and it showed. As "Skipper," he tried to fly every day and his instructor pilots respected him for "staying in the pits."

Yes, it's true, the "Texas Riviera," as Corpus Christi is known by the locals, is a fairly remote location on the Gulf Coast, but Peggy and I loved it. Since we had lived in "Corpus" four years earlier when I had been a student pilot, we felt comfortable with the area and settled right in. We bought a house that backed up to a salt-water canal on historic Padre Island National Seashore. We enjoyed fishing from our back porch and laughing hysterically as Scooter, all three pounds of her, "fished" along with us. The moment she saw the tips of our fishing poles jerk down she would jump off our dock into the water after our catch. The fish usually outweighed her. We'd sit out there with the sun on our backs, the wind in our faces and Navy trainers doing acrobatics above our heads. I'd think about airplanes, Peggy would think about babies (and our lack of them), and Scooter would think about "the one that got away."

On weekends I flew a Pterodactyl, an ultralight aircraft that I bought secondhand at a garage sale for $1500—no questions asked. The 'dactyl was basically a beefed up hang glider with a propeller driven tricycle frame hanging beneath it. A forward wing, called a canard, made it virtually stall proof and gave it a top speed of about 55 mph. I put it together and flew it on the beaches of Padre Island with the help of a friend, Leon McJunkin.

Leon was a 65-year-old weight lifter who looked about 35. I remember Leon's wife once commenting to me, "You should have seen how young he looked before the accident." Leon had been involved in a midair collision between two ultralights five years earlier and fell a couple of hundred feet straight down onto the beach. After being released from the hospital several months later, Leon no longer flew ultralights. But his expertise and encouragement to other ultralight pilots, especially Pterodactyl pilots like me, was without equal.

WHAM!
Goss Steals Airplane—By Mistake

I had been fascinated with the Pterodactyl ever since I accidently flew one in Maine. After taking a float plane lesson on the Kennebec River, I watched a guy land a tiny, colorful, lightweight aircraft in a nearby field. I walked up and said hello. Not ever having seen me before, he asked if I wanted to try taxiing this new fangled thing around on the grass. "Sure," I said with a grin. Moments later, a strong crosswind lifted me skyward pushing my flight path sideways and directly into a large tree. With a choice of crashing or flying, I chose the later. I powered over the tree and flew around for ten minutes as I tried to figure out what to do next and basically watched the owner on the ground have a conniption fit.

My first attempt at landing had too high a sink rate as I tried to land near the feet of the distraught owner, so I had to execute a go around. The upset owner knew that if I wanted to fly his $10,000 investment fifty miles away and land—or crash—it was now completely out of his control. Foolishly, he had passed control of his aircraft to a total stranger. He wasn't as big an idiot as I was, though. I had accepted his offer without the foggiest notion of how to fly the 'dactyl because the rear engine propeller and the front canard gave this aircraft flying characteristics completely different to anything I had ever flown before. In most airplanes, when you add power with the throttle, the pilot gets an almost instantaneous "seat of the pants" sensation of climbing, and when power is reduced, a sense of descent. However, as I discovered, the forward canard and pusher propeller of the Pterodactyl created a reversal of that seat of the pants sensation. For the first few seconds after I added power (an ungodly long amount of time in an airplane under many circumstances), I felt an immediate rate of descent, not ascent. I sensed it with both my peripheral vision and my butt, which also happened to be the location of my brain at this particular moment in time. I was scared, but also having a helluva great time. It was then and there that I decided, if I survived, I'd buy my own Pterodactyl someday. What a wild ride!

My next approach for landing was flatter, safer and in no way resembled my earlier approach when I gave the poor guy on the ground the impression that I was trying to behead him with the left wing. When I smoothly touched down, no worse for the wear, he ran over to me white faced and said, "I thought you were a goner—praise the Lord." He was one happy camper. As it turned out, I was lucky to have landed when I did. As I helped him disassemble his ultralight and put it in the back of his station wagon an ugly thunderstorm blew into the area and nearly blew the place off the map.

One evening, after Peggy and I arrived home from the "World Famous San Patricio Rattlesnake Races" (I took second place, losing by a nose—I mean snout) I heard a loud buzzing as we stepped from the car into the garage. It sounded like a rattlesnake. Finally, I noticed this huge June bug banging against the florescent light over my workbench. Snatching it from the air with my left hand, I realized it was a tiny hummingbird.

"Hummer" became a guest in our house for a few weeks as we fed it nectar to help it regain its strength. What a dynamite little flyer. Moving his wings at over seventy beats per second, he could fly backward, forward or remain perfectly stationary in flight as he fed from the sugar water feeder we hung from a light in the center of our guest bedroom ceiling. He was as cute as he was courageous, defending his feeder like a sow bear with cubs. Soon, the little green firecracker was ready for release.

Peg and I took him outside into the ever-blowing Corpus Christi wind and I uncupped my hands. He sat there for a moment, quizzically looking at us before he took off. Up he went, straight up over our heads directly into the noonday sun. I kept watching him as he climbed like a Trident missile, the strongly blowing hot wind causing no deviation in his upward flight. Finally, thousands of feet above us, Hummer disappeared into the sun—still directly and perfectly overhead. How and why that little sucker went straight up I'll never know, but I'd like to, from a strictly aeronautical point of view. Hummer's flying ability had been a wonder to behold!

Living on Padre Island National Seashore was a naturalist's dream. A favorite event of my Aunt Fran and ours was the seasonal baby sea turtle release. Assisting a National Seashore naturalist, we would follow newly hatched Ridley sea turtles, a rare species, down into the ocean. Then we'd scoop them up with a net and return the adorable little hatchlings to the naturalist who then raised them to a larger size. Once imprinted by that first swim, an extra year's growth in captivity would help to protect them from predators. They would be released during the following year's hatch as older, stronger, bigger and possibly wiser yearlings, which would help ensure the survival of a rapidly diminishing species. Because of their initial imprinting from nearby ocean water after they hatched, many of these same turtles would return to Padre Island years later as adults to nest, replenishing the local population of this rare and beautiful creature of the seas. Peg and I have always felt an obligation to help preserve the God-given natural diversity with which Earth has been so fortunately blessed. The way I figured it, once a species is gone, it's gone for good, and it will take the overturning of Heaven and Hell before we see the uniqueness of that creature again. So, we've just got to help out Mother Nature the best we can.

CHAPTER SEVEN

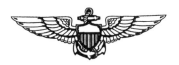

WHAM!
AND THEN THERE WERE FOUR

After a year of strikeouts in the pregnancy department, Peg and I met with some fertility doctors. We started on their protocol of "totally spontaneous love making"—as long as it was on a certain day of the month, at a certain time of day, before a bath, but after a light snack, well you know what I mean, SPONTANEOUS. I vaguely remember Doctor Caceres talking about some kind of malfunctioning egg releasing thing and further "egg adhering difficulties" stuff. And all these years I had thought that sex was simple and uncomplicated!

One night, Peg and I were driving from the airport when a car ran a stop sign on a remote rain-covered stretch of highway. I knew there was no way to stop on the slick highway as Peggy opened her weary eyes to see the side of a stalled car rapidly approaching our car's windshield. To me, it was a shocking reminder of the visual picture I had of the Air Force A-10s closing in on my P-3 Orion at over 700 miles per hour. Bug-eyed, Peggy screamed as we both realized my shot at passing behind the now-stalled car was gone. Certain we were going to die in an absolutely gruesome car crash, I snapped the wheel to the right and prayed that the stopped car wouldn't move forward into our path. Terrified, we listened for the tell-tale sounds of screeching metal on metal as I saw the enormous moon-sized eyes of the stalled driver whip by my left eye's peripheral vision. Whew, no scratching metal sounds! But a concrete telephone pole was rushing up to greet the front of our little car. I gently tried to ease the steering wheel back to the left, fully aware that the tires would be unable to maintain their grip on the slick cement highway much longer. And then...POP...all tire friction with the road was gone and control of the car was no longer in my hands. From my flight training I knew we were now hydroplaning. As we started spinning down that wet road, Peg and I screamed in terrified unison. We twirled, like a high-speed centrifuge, eight times before coming to rest in the deep rain soaked mud of the highway median. "Peg, are...are...are you okay?" I said in utter amazement that we weren't dead.

"I th...th...think so," she mumbled.

"Good, 'cuz I'm gonna kill that stupid idiot!" I screamed as I jumped out of the car into the knee-deep mud while hearing the engine of the stalled car struggle and suddenly come roaring to life. As it started to pull away, I dove through the driver's side window like a mud covered maniac and yanked the keys from the ignition, ending all hopes for the idiot's escape. I was so damn mad I could have backed a bulldog off a plate of guts, and the very sleepy driver sobered up quickly. An enormous, very confused looking guy emerged from the car and sheepishly asked me for his keys.

When the police finally showed up, they made me return his keys. Peg and I were left stuck in the mud, abandoned by both the jerk who almost killed us and the police who nearly cited me with disturbing the peace. That threat particularly perturbed me because there was no one on that stretch of rural highway to disturb except the policeman and the idiot. They just happened to be on a first name basis.

As we arrived home early that morning, exhausted and covered in mud, Peggy reminded me of the "to the minute" schedule our fertility specialist recommended. "You've got to be kidding me," was all I could mumble. The schedule had so far proven worthless and we were both so tired we couldn't see, or anything else, straight—but, what the hell. Butta-Bing, Butta-Bang, Butta-Boom, sleep....

Counting back the days, I'm still convinced that it was the gut wrenching primal screaming of the near collision that had slung an egg, like a spermatozoan TOA, or target of opportunity, (more pilot talk) into the innermost confines of my adorable wife. That wild ride did the trick! It was just what the doctor ordered. I reflected on Doc Caceres's previous "this releasing" and "that adhering" sex stuff discussions. It was a trick delivered to us by an angel: the enormous, moon-eyed, disguised like an idiot, Angel of Highway 37. Throw away the thermometer—Peggy was finally pregnant.

I'll never forget the sonogram technician's startled exclamation, "Oh my goodness!" as she looked at the TV monitor while she glided the sono-transmitter across Peggy's rapidly expanding torso four months later. I began to feel ill. Every time the technician would mumble "Oh my goodness" I'd look at the monitor and see a two-headed baby. Suddenly I became so brokenhearted—but I had to be careful not to upset Peggy. I used to harangue my flight students with the torturously old cliche "two heads are better than one" to reinforce the importance of crew coordination. "I promise I will never use another cliche as long as I live...." I prayed as I held Peggy's hand and again peeked over my shoulder at the two-headed monster on the screen. I was paralyzed, horrified, mortified, all the while doing my best to keep a cheerful smile on my face for Peggy, who squeezed my hand and then flashed me her beautiful smile. Flat on her back, she didn't have a good view of the monitor, clueless to my torment and the horror she held within.

When the doctor finally entered the room and announced we were having twins—independent of one another—I jumped for joy in the knowledge that with the two heads came two distinct bodies. From the juxtapositional view on the monitor that I had seen, it seemed like a miracle to me. Two eggs—not one—had been flung from Peg's ovaries that fateful night. I laughed hysterically at the news; I was so relieved. Peggy cried. Women do that sometimes.

We called to tell Pop, my 97-year-old World War I aviator

granddad, that Peggy was pregnant with twins. He commented "Oh, that's nice—I had twin brothers."

"You did, Pop?" Peggy happily remarked at the coincidence.

"Yeah, they both died at birth." He stated matter-of-factly. I guess after you'd lived as long as Pop had lived, life no longer offered any surprises—or required any tactfulness.

In the future, when people would ask if twins ran in our family, my answer became "Well yeah...kind of...."

After Peggy became pregnant, we decided that, as a new father-to-be, I'd have to start settling down. I put the Pterodactyl up for sale in the *Corpus Christi Caller Times*. A stranger showed up, quickly paid me the $1700 asking price, (I thought he'd bargain me down) packed it up in the back of his truck and drove off—no questions asked. I was flabbergasted. The cycle began anew, I'm sure, with that guy suddenly 100 feet in the air, at the controls of that fool thing, looking to all the world like ET bicycling above the moonlit countryside, saying to himself, "What the hell do I do now?"

One day, while I was conducting Basic Instrument training, which we called BIs, over the Gulf of Mexico, I received a subtle message over the base radio frequency, "Goss, her water broke, RTB...." (more pilot talk meaning "Return to Base.") I put the T-44 into a steep dive and landed in no time flat. Sprinting to my car, I left my white-knuckled student behind to secure the plane.

"This was happening a little bit early," I thought. "But, Peggy's tummy is e-e-e-enormous." More beautiful than ever, I still couldn't understand how Peggy could get out of bed, no less walk and exercise like everything was status quo. I wondered if Peggy's gardening that morning had been such a good idea after all.

That night, I was there to help with the delivery of Brian and Christie. It was the most incredible moment and the most awesome gift from God that Peggy and I will ever receive—the gift of two beautiful, healthy babies. Thanks, Doc Caceres, wherever you are. You were the greatest—even though I couldn't understand a damn word you said half the time. The devotion you demonstrated to your patients with your heart said it all.

As our three year tour in Corpus Christi came to an end, we put our house up for rent and prepared for another move—this time to Naval Air Station Alemeda, just outside San Francisco. Before we left, I completed my MBA on the campus of Corpus Christi State University. There I often found western diamondback rattlesnakes parked under my old Volvo Amazon after night classes. Apparently, the warmth of its engine attracted the rattlers on the cooler nights. I quickly learned to look under the Amazon before stepping in. Soon we would be leaving the wild, wild, west—a place both Peggy and I had grown to love.

As the time to leave grew near, a couple of the local Commanding Officers somehow lined me up for one of the most prestigious—and difficult—jobs a Navy lieutenant can get. I would be Assistant Navigator of USS *Carl Vinson*, a giant nuclear aircraft carrier. This was going to be sea duty, the real McCoy, and it wasn't supposed to be a good time. Soon our fun filled little world of planes, babies and fish would be blown to smithereens—we just didn't know it yet.

I read about it in the base library only a few weeks before—the USS *Carl Vinson*. Now here it was floating before me—one of the world's largest man-made gray things—a Nimitz class nuclear aircraft carrier. By far the biggest, baddest, most complex weapons platform ever built, with a range of over one million miles between refuelings, a Nimitz class carrier is vastly more capable in speed, endurance, maneuvering and carrying capacity than anything ever built before them.

Forming the centerpiece of the Carrier Battle Group and

America's naval strategy, the *Vinson* was both a national treasure and a showpiece valued at several billion dollars just in hardware alone. A monstrous, high-speed, all-purpose floating airport, home to a hundred tactical jet aircraft of various sorts, a person needs to see it to believe the immensity of it. It is the aircraft carrier's ability to launch and recover aircraft that sets it apart from all the other ships of the world. Without this unique capability a giant carrier is "like a cruise ship without a pool."

As I looked, transfixed at the *Carl Vinson* for the first time, never did it occur to me that, in less than a year I'd be high up in the Navigation Bridge, serving as the Officer of the Deck, steaming along at greater than 25 knots into the dark Pacific Ocean. I would be entrusted by the Captain with complete and full responsibility for this supremely capable nuclear behemoth. If the image had not been simply incomprehensible, it undoubtedly would have been utterly terrifying. But, I've gotten ahead of myself.

From Corpus Christi, Peg, the twins, Scooter and I drove to San Diego where I attended a few months of navigation, boat handling and shipboard fire-fighting school. Navigation school was hard as hell but fire-fighting school was even harder. We ran into horizontally placed towering infernos ablaze with huge oil fed fires with powerful water hoses and special asbestos clothing. We practiced and practiced rescues and different fire-fighting techniques until we got it right. A raging fire on a ship in the open ocean is a sailor's worst nightmare. There are not a lot of options. If you don't put the fire out then you are either going to burn, suffocate or drown. We trained to be self-sufficient. We trained to keep the ship afloat at all costs. We trained to work as a team. We trained to survive.

Later, I came to discover that a ship the size of the *Vinson*—1100-feet long, 250-feet wide, higher than a 24-story building, longer than the Empire State Building, weighing close to 100,000 tons, with over 5000 young men and women on board—had fires break out on it almost every day. I understood why the fire-fighting school had to be so realistic. It was because we

Pavlov's dog, I would respond as fast as possible to that
trying hard to give Peggy a break from the kids during
es when the ship was at the pier. The twins were being potty
ied and if we were not quick enough to assist, the little
gers would revert back to crapping in their diapers in no
flat. "So, this is what being a parent is all about," I thought
flinched at another plaintiff "WIPE!" that pierced the si-
e. I reflected on my beautiful wife, Peggy, who was out
shopping. How was she going to handle toilet training
toddlers, alone, for months on end? It was going to be
ire. I felt bad about leaving her so often and for so long, but
is one of the sacrifices that military people and their fami-
leal with constantly.

f it hadn't been for my unique sense of humor, I swear I
ld have come apart at the seams. I almost did at times. The
nsibilities I had as a devoted, loving, new father of twin
ers and those as the Captain and Navigator's professional
ything" man were completely at odds. What I needed was
id and twin me's not one me and twin kids.

eggy was not getting a big kick out of life in Northern
ornia. At least not the kind of "kick" I told her she'd get.
wins never gave her a chance. Plus, she couldn't get used
e cold after having lived in Texas. Mark Twain once
ed, "The coldest winter I ever spent was my summer in
rancisco." Peggy, who had to keep the kids in sweaters
ghout the summer, didn't think it was such a big joke.

lear aircraft carrier is a world showcase, ready to employ
ver and prestige anywhere in the world as directed by the
lent of the United States. One of my jobs was to ceremo-
coordinate getting civilian and military VIP's safely off
ngerous flight deck, usually after they had made their
resting gear landing. With decelerations of 150 knots to
second or less, it was much more like a controlled crash
"landing." Stunned, confused, exhilarated and airsick,

fought shipboard fires routinely. While I
emergency fire parties we ordered over the
various parts of the ship to fight fires never
fully, most of the fires they found were smal
start small.

After completing the required courses in S
up to San Francisco and rented a little hou
land, in Alameda, near the Navy Base. I t
settle into our new "home" with Brian and
thirteen months old at the time, but I knev
be flying to Subic Bay, Philippines, to joi
relieve the present Assistant Navigator of h
sibilities. This tour of duty would be exce
Peggy. I was worried for her. Depression
was a fact of life among many of the sailors
was going to be a very challenging enviro
on the ship.

In the meantime, I would help Peggy
sible during the brief periods I was hom
time father like Peggy was a first time mo
was going to take some practice for both

The accident in Spain had been a traumatic
he had recovered remarkably well from it
accolades while an instructor pilot in Trai
One. When they offered him the extremely s
job of Assistant Navigator on a nuclear aircr
for him but secretly nervous as well. In the
jobs are usually very hard jobs and as a
wondered how we were going to manage.

Parenthood—what a trip! I remember
room at the sound of a plaintiff wail, '

were just a few of the "arresting expressions" I detected from our arriving guests. Board chairmen and CEOs of giant Fortune 500 companies were constantly riding the ship as guests of the U.S. Government via the Captain.

The CEO of Sony Electronics, Mr. Morita, was one such VIP who I helped to escort around the ship for a few days until he flew off. A day later, I handed the Captain an article from a *US News and World Report* magazine stating that Morita, the Sony CEO, had published a book brutally critical of America. The book attacked its work ethic and lack of high technological capabilities. Captain Borchers just shook his head after reading it. The *Vinson's* guest list for its VIP program was sometimes unusual.

Another time we had a huge celebrity lunch in the ship's enormous hangar bay for the American Academy of Achievement. This was a bizarre grouping of super achieving celebrities and businessmen with a select group of super achieving high school seniors. One naval officer was assigned per table. We were dressed in our tropical white uniform, serving as kind of a table conversation piece for the celebrities. It really was a great deal, though, because the food was good and it was fun to "scope out" all the notables and celebrities and to listen to them pontificate at the podium. I thought the best speaker of the day was Oprah Winfrey and the worst was Tom Clancy, whose speech made him sound like he had been a military hero instead of the gifted writer that he is.

I sat between Arthur Rock, venture capitalist behind the Intel Corporation, and Ralph Lauren, the world famous clothes designer who turned out to be a great guy. At the next table over were Steven Spielburg, George Lucas and General Colin Powell. Beverly Sills, Tom Selleck and Earnest and Julius Gallo, the vineyard magnates, sat at the table beyond. The list of celebrities and billionaires went on and on.

But, the biggest surprise of all was that the king of junk bonds, Mike Milken, appeared to be the honored guest at this gathering. He was even given a brand new leather flight jacket which he proudly wore along with his toupee. It struck me as odd that he was an honored guest on our nation's most prestigious warship even though he was under investigation for a whole slew of Securities and Exchange violations by the U.S. Government—violations that cost U.S. taxpayers and pensioners billions upon billions of dollars. Mike asked me what I did on the ship and I told him I assisted the Captain and the Navigator on the Bridge. He immediately retorted "Well, I want you to know that I'm financing a ship bigger than this next week!"

"Well, excuuseee me, but I—don't—think—so." I thought to myself.

I figured he had an ego big enough to be a fighter jock, although his eyes had to be worn out from counting all his money. I'd read that he had "earned" $1.8 billion over a three-year period. I laughed to myself as I shook hands with him and smiled for a picture. My oldest brother, Bob, and I had worked together in high school as garbage men. Bob had taken those skills and was now a successful bond salesman on Wall Street. I sent him a photograph. It was of Milken and me shaking hands, me in uniform, each with a big toothy grin on our faces. Below the picture, I jokingly placed a caption that I knew my brother would enjoy. It read, "Junk Bond King Mike Milken and Lt. Bill Goss have just completed the sale of the United States Navy to Japan."

Big Bob keeps that picture on his desk for use as an icebreaker during business meetings, unless it's a meeting with the SEC. He and I look a little too much alike for them to get the humor of it.

Lately I heard that Milken had been diagnosed with prostate cancer and successfully beat it. Since his challenges with incarceration and cancer, he has contributed vast amounts of time and money as a leader in the fight against prostate cancer. I think that's fantastic. He now must realize money can't buy happiness even when you have billions at your disposal. To paraphrase the Good Book, "What's the gain if you gain the whole world but lose your soul?"

While steaming around the globe I often went without any significant sleep for days because the workload was so high. During the rare free time that I didn't use to study for my Officer of the Deck qualifications or to catch up on sleep, I let off steam by rolling out wrestling mats beneath the wings of F-14 Tomcat fighter jets. I wrestled or boxed with other sailors in an enormous aircraft maintenance hangar just below the flight deck. It was an unusual gymnasium setting, under the wings of F-14s, with puddles of hydraulic fluid and heavy tie-down chains all over the place. But to the sailors and U.S. Marines aboard a naval combatant at sea, improvisation, whether for work, physical fitness or folly, will always be the name of the game.

I was held accountable for the equipment on the Navigation Bridge during my tour of duty on *Carl Vinson*. My greatest fear was that someone would steal the two-pound cast aluminum steering wheel thus rendering this multi-billion dollar national asset incapable of fulfilling commitments during an international crisis. And as crazy as this may seem, this extremely annoying thing happened twice causing more than a few fitful nights. A few days before we were to get underway for a two-week workup cruise, I was looking over the bridge console, or "the helm" as it is known in sailor lingo, and I noticed the ship's steering wheel was missing.

"Chief, where's the steering wheel?" I queried.

"I have no idea, Lieutenant Goss," was his alarmed reply.

To make a long story short, someone unscrewed this little 12-inch diameter cast aluminum steering wheel and took it home as a souvenir. For good. The end. We had a multi-billion dollar ship with no way to drive it, if you can believe it. We finally ended up jury-rigging some kind of wheel to the console to get us through that two-week cruise. I ordered a couple of steering wheels like the one that had come with the ship. They were very expensive for only a couple pounds of cheap cast metal, but fulfilled a much more important role than the infamous six hundred dollar toilet seat like the one found on the P-3 Orion.

During the ordering process, the makeshift steering wheel was stolen as well.

Thankfully, the new steering wheels arrived just before we were expected to get underway again. It was a nerve-racking ordeal for me, though I'm certain it must have provided someone a laugh. Nobody wants to tell the Chief of Naval Operations, or the Secretary of Defense or the President of the United States, that one of our nation's nuclear aircraft carriers can't get underway because someone stole the steering wheel. The policy for the new steering wheels was that they were to be kept under lock and key in the Captain's safe when not actually being used to drive the ship.

During a two month long Pacific Rim Exercise called PACEX, the first few weeks consisted of NLOA which was an acronym for "Near Land Operating Areas" procedures. This was pretty wild stuff and involved driving this humongous ship into tiny natural harbors surrounded by the small mountainous islands of the Aleutians off the coast of Alaska. The idea was that the ship could remain undetected by the enemy due to the tall mountains hiding or masking the large radar signature of the ship. The problem was that in order to conduct flight operations the ship normally had to run in a kind of race track pattern, one leg into the wind for launches and recoveries and one leg against the wind to get back to the starting point or to cover ground in order to get to the destination. In near land operating scenarios we could be steaming the ship toward a mountain and be forced to turn out of the wind prior to recovering all the aircraft due to the lack of maneuvering space. Also the fog and heavy seas common to coastal Alaska caused a constant threat of grounding or colliding with a mountain, where in the open ocean such a risk is nearly nonexistent. This all translated into "no sleep" for the navigation team until we reached "Blue Water" or open ocean operations once again.

After departing the Aleutian Islands four exhausting days later, we went right into an underway replenishment evolution. This tricky maneuver involved the aircraft carrier steaming up alongside a much smaller oiler or freighter while cruising at 10-15 knots. Once stabilized, lines were shot across each other's decks pulling cables to ultimately connect huge oil hoses between the ships for the transfer of thousands of gallons of aviation fuel, as well as food, equipment, bombs, and personnel. The goal was for the aircraft carrier to maintain constant relative position to the other ship (approximately 120 feet of water separation in between). This is done while flight ops were being conducted, in heavy seas, and while turning to avoid collision with a right of way ship, and so forth. It usually worked. Sometimes things didn't go so well.

Once, we lost control of our rudder during an underway replenishment. Someone had inadvertently shut off one of the huge hydraulic pumps that powered the rudder system. We started veering into the 700-foot long replenishment ship as the conning officer barked out orders to no avail in an attempt to increase separation. The Captain jumped in and took over the conn. When we were within 80 feet of the other ship and closing fast, he ordered "Emergency Breakaway, Emergency Breakaway." This dangerous emergency procedure was the last ditch effort to avoid a potentially deadly collision between the two ships.

Immediately, the massive fuel transfer hoses that straddled between the two ships were broken, spraying highly pressurized jet fuel all over the ships, personnel and the sea. The replenishment vessel, which normally was responsible for maintaining a steady course, now attempted to maneuver to starboard to open distance from the malfunctioning aircraft carrier. In this particular instance we got within forty feet of one another before we started opening the space between us again. It was a very close call. Lives were at stake and the Captain's career was on the line.

Within a few minutes the Captain and the crew had forgotten all about it, hard at work at some new task. That is the nature of life on board an aircraft carrier—always trying to stay one step ahead of catastrophe—always too much work at hand to dwell on any given close calls. Although the guilty party was almost always sought out and disciplined, the pressing work schedule forced the theme, "Keep moving forward and get the job done."

During PACEX (which involved several other battle groups and numerous other ships and submarines), the Admirals got together and united us into a giant diamond formation of seventy ships. It was the largest peacetime formation of ships since WWII. F-14 Tomcats flew overhead and snapped pictures while the radar screen in the Combat Information Center (CIC) looked like a giant constellation of blinking stars. It was an impressive sight seeing all those aircraft carriers and battleships leading the group. They were damn big blips. The E-2 Hawkeye early warning aircraft orbited above the ship and transmitted a great radar picture down to us.

While in the Sea of Japan during very high wave conditions, we lost a man overboard. It is probable he had taken a smoke break in an area where personnel were forbidden to enter during high sea activity. From out of nowhere, an exceptionally large wave, a "rogue" wave as they are referred, came along and swept him right off the ship. Unfortunately, the two guys he was with didn't tell anyone up on the bridge until they had spent half-an-hour looking for him "thinking that he had somehow gotten inside." Since we, and the battle group behind us, had been steaming ahead at 26 knots at the time, we had already covered thirteen nautical miles since the estimated time he washed overboard. Also the sun had begun to set by this time as well. The poor guy was in a very bad way. But the Captain and the Admiral ordered the entire battle group and its aircraft to look for this young sailor for two days. I was on the bridge using night vision goggles hoping to pick up an infrared signal from his body heat. But he was gone. It was something to see: billions of dollars worth of assets being used by thousands of men and women as they searched for one U.S. sailor who didn't have a chance in hell of being alive. It made me feel proud. Yet, it also struck me as ironic that after all I had been through, this young sailor was swept away in an instant by an enormous wave coming out of nowhere. Fate and destiny are sometimes hard to understand.

Soon after that we got word that an earthquake, a really big one, had struck in San Francisco. It was terribly demoralizing news for the crew because, being at sea, we were without access to a telephone to check on our family's welfare. We knew we'd have to wait for another week until we pulled into Pusan, Korea before calling home. One officer was summoned to the bridge to see the Captain. A few hours later he was flown off the ship to make plans for his wife's funeral. She had been in a commuter van on the second deck of the Oakland Bay Bridge when the top deck collapsed, crushing all the cars beneath it. It was devastating news. Besides feeling sorrow for the officer who lost his wife, everyone kept wondering how their loved ones fared as well.

When we got to Pusan, I finally got Peggy on the hotel phone. She and the kids had been terrified. The earthquake had made a sound like the crack of a rifle that echoed throughout the neighborhood while knocking them to the floor. The kids cried when the hanging light fixtures crashed back and forth into each side of the ceiling. Luckily the houses in our immediate neighborhood were spared heavy damage but many within the San Francisco Bay area were totally destroyed.

On sailing back into San Francisco three weeks later, we had to have newly surveyed bottom contour charts sent to us. Not only was our usual clearance under the Oakland Bay Bridge by inches (after we lowered our highest mast, we were still just under 200 feet high) but normally we had only a few feet of clearance beneath our 38-foot keel depth at high tide. If certain parts of the ocean floor had risen during the quake even by a foot or two, we ran the risk of grounding the ship. Luckily the new survey established that we had just enough clearance both below and above the ship for a safe return. When we passed beneath the Golden Gate Bridge, I was first struck by how few wind surfers were out on the bay. Normally there'd be hundreds of them in front of us like colorful butterflies. They would dart across our bow like suicidal Kamakaze pilots while we steamed forward in the heavy current at 15 knots, completely unable to prevent running over anybody if they capsized their windsurfer in front of us. As we passed between Alcatraz and downtown San Francisco, we could see the charred and broken remains of some previously beautiful homes and buildings. In the distance stood the Oakland Bay Bridge with its top deck still collapsed. Our berth lay just a few miles beyond it in the ship turning basin.

Reunion at home was both wonderful and bittersweet. Our families all knew we'd be leaving again real soon—and that's a lousy feeling, I've got to tell you. Still, we all tried to make the most of our time together.

In no time at all we were on the high seas again, at the start of a six month deployment. One particularly beautiful day in the middle of the Pacific Ocean I was giving Captain Borchers a position report on some distant ship traffic when a tremendous "Kaabooom" rocked the ship, momentarily causing the entire vessel to pop down and up from the enormous compression of the explosion. Doyle Borchers, was nearly knocked out of his comfortable perch in the Captain's Chair, and I was mystified as we watched window glass blow out of a helicopter parked below us. I thought we had either hit a mine or had been torpedoed. The Captain's phone immediately rang. "Well, gosh darn it (not really what he said), don't ever let that happen again without clearance from me first," he said as he slammed the receiver down into the Air Operations Officer's ear. Captain Borchers, being a F-14 pilot himself, turned, smiled approvingly at me and said, "A Tomcat just broke the sound barrier above the ship—did you see it go by?"

"No sir," I said, "but I think I heard it."

Shortly after that, while in the Sea of Japan, hundreds of ships' position lights were scattered in constant random movement in front of us in the otherwise total darkness. It was a gigantic fleet of Japanese fishing trawlers on top of some prime fishing waters. We were proceeding along at a fast 25 knots to arrive at our destination in time for high tide. I had to keep waking the Captain up to give him contact reports of how close other ships were, in accordance with his standing orders. As the number of ship contacts grew larger, it was rapidly becoming an out-of-control situation. International Maritime Rules of the Road are generally applicable for two ships encountering one another alone on the high seas, not for hundreds of ships, many of which ignored or didn't understand the rules anyway.

During that midwatch, what I believed to be a midsized Japanese trawler in the black night kept driving right toward *Carl Vinson's* bow regardless of our maneuvering. I had to ask the Captain out onto the bridge at 3 o'clock in the morning. He got there just in time to see this other ship disappear into the "shadow zone" of our ship, which is 566 yards of ocean area in front of the bow that cannot be seen from the navigation bridge. I ordered the aircraft carrier into a hard port turn and was about to sound the tremendously loud blast of the collision alarm when the Captain, the rest of the bridge team and I saw the running lights of this trawler pass very close to the starboard side. The trawler, probably curious as to our unusual lighting scene, had simply sailed towards us to take a look. They must have shit sushi when they discovered that they had placed themselves directly in the path of an enormous aircraft carrier running close to top speed. An exhausted Captain Borchers, almost too tired to care, looked at me and said politely, "Good job, ANAV. Well...good night."

WHAM!
"BOOOOM!"

One afternoon, toward the end of my tour of duty, I had just assumed the duties and responsibilities as the underway Officer of the Deck (OOD) in the stormy Pacific during flight operations. I was breaking in my newly aboard relief, Assistant Navigator Lieutenant Frank Gren. Smart, funny and cocky, he stated, "Bill, this OOD stuff looks easy—nothing ever happens up here—I can take it from here."

At that moment an F-14 pilot trying to touchdown aborted the landing and inadvertently rocked his wings to the right at the moment he went to full afterburner. That caused the Tomcat to move approximately ten feet to the right of the safe landing zone. A split second later, "BOOOOM!" his right wing tip contacted the tail of a parked A-7 Corsair, a light attack jet. The contact destroyed that aircraft and blew shrapnel, like silver confetti, up into the very thick glass windows of the navigation bridge, behind which Commander Mantei, Lt. Frank Gren and I stood with our jaws to the floor. For a brief moment in time, the airborne F-14, now missing several feet of its starboard wing tip and dramatically slowed down by the impact, appeared to be virtually standing still on its tail in full afterburner just feet above the carrier deck and immediately off the bow. I prayed real quick that the Tomcat wouldn't stall out and fall back onto the flight deck crowded with hundreds of crewmen and dozens of jets full of fuel. The explosion and fire would have been devastating. Time, for that brief moment, seemed to stand still.

After what seemed like an eternity but in reality was just seconds, the stupendous power of the F-14 Tomcat's engines started to inch it shakily skyward. Finally the badly shaken pilot and his RIO (Radar Intercept Officer) began another approach from the holding pattern above the ship, and this one thankfully resulted in a safe trap.

Immediately after the collision, I looked at the ship's compass. It was almost perfectly steady in the rough seas. I had the quartermaster log the ships heading as steady on 275 plus or minus one degree because my past experiences told me that this information would prove to be vital at a future date. After the damaged F-14 landed safely, I finally turned to Lt. Gren and responded, "Yeah, this OOD stuff is easy—nothing ever happens—you can take it from here."

A month later, the Navigator, Commander Bob Mantei, told me the F-14 squadron's Accident Investigation Board was trying to pin the blame on the Navigation Department for having the ship in a turn or not holding the ship's heading steady for the landing. Bob was an extremely competent "Gator" and a wonderful leader and friend. I told him not to worry. He looked up from the ship's logbook after reading it and just smiled. It was a smile of relief, knowing one more fire had been put out. And that was the last we ever heard about that accident.

On one particularly stress-filled visit home, I jokingly said to Peggy, "You're mean to me, you don't like me anymore."

Without skipping a beat, she responded quickly, "Oh, don't feel bad, Bill. I never liked you." What a great sense of humor... I think. It was definitely time for a change of scenery—for all of us.

As the result of my tour of duty on the USS *Carl Vinson*, I was awarded a Navy Commendation Medal for the work I had done. Lord knows I didn't deserve it. But, for the Assistant Navigator of a nuclear carrier, if the ship is kept from running aground or having a collision at sea, a medal is automatic. Plus, the Captain's kind wife, Jeanne, thought I was nice, and that never hurt anything.

I had asked Peggy where she wanted to go for our next tour of duty and she gave me that stony-eyed "you've got to be kidding me" look. Finally she responded, "To Jacksonville, Florida, where the kids can wear T-shirts and shorts year round." Thanks to a great Navy Assignments Officer in Washington, D.C, we were on our way to Jacksonville a few months later. As we drove away from our little rental house and down our neighborhood street for the last time, I watched for some kind of sign that Peggy might miss that place. She never looked back.

What can I say about Bill's tour of duty in California? For starters, I hated it with a passion. We moved from a spacious, warm place where we had lots of friends, to a tiny cold spot. We had frost on our breath every morning and we didn't know anybody. Plus, as a new mother of twin toddlers, I needed help and emotional support and Bill was always at sea.

I married Bill; I didn't marry the Navy. Although I'm certain Bill would disagree, the sacrifice the Navy asks of dependents—as they call us—is sometimes just too much. It's the only job I know where husbands are routinely expected to leave their wives and children for six months at a time with no resources for making phone calls and with lengthy delays in the mail service. It's really rough on the kids too. Everybody misses Dad and no one, including me, knows why he has to be gone so long. It was just so hard to understand. Although life as a Navy wife was challenging, it was later events beyond the realm of Bill's military career that proved to be the greatest challenges of our future.

Part Two

Insights

After the Fall

"Although change and adversity can cause great stress,
Persevere and don't fret at your lack of success,
Because success is failure turned inside out—
The silver tint in the clouds of doubt,
And you never can tell just how close you are,
It may be near when it seems so far;
So stick to the fight when you're hardest hit—
It's when things seem worst that you must not quit."
—Anonymous

"He who has a why to live
can bear with any how."
— Nietzche

CHAPTER EIGHT

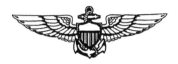

WHAM!
GOSS LOGS FLIGHT TIME—
WITHOUT AN AIRPLANE

T he trip from San Francisco to Jacksonville, Florida, was a happy one for Peggy and me. Called "Jax" by the locals and home to the newest NFL expansion team, the Jacksonville Jaguars, we had a pretty house on a heavily wooded lot just off the St. John's River. Peg and I had bought it the month before on a frantic "time is running out" weekend house hunting trip.

"Everything is going to be perfect from now on," I voiced to Peggy. She just gave me that famous smile of hers that indicates she knows I'm eternally optimistic but she doesn't believe a word I'm saying.

We had been in Jacksonville about a year and it was my last day as Training Officer when I was driving home on Interstate 295 one day for lunch. I was really looking forward to starting a refresher flight training curriculum to fly the P-3C Orion as a senior pilot and Squadron Department Head.

Suddenly, I noticed cars ahead of me swerving to avoid hitting something in the road. It appeared to be a large box of garbage smack in the middle of the two southbound lanes. I slowed as I approached this big carton of trash. The traffic around me was light, with gorgeous driving conditions and great visibility. Dad used to tell me, "Bill, never drive past something in the road that could hurt the driver behind you. Do the right thing." It was another E. J. Goss credo, echoing in my head as I saw the car in front of me swerve to avoid hitting the box.

"Gotta do it," I said as I pulled off the right side of the highway onto the grass. When the coast was clear, I trotted across the highway and grabbed the carton, pulling it into the middle of a 100-foot wide grass covered median. Feeling like the Good Samaritan, I watched cars now proceed safely and unobstructed down the interstate. I remained standing in the center of the lush grass median looking for a large space between the oncoming cars in the distance as I planned my careful return to the other side of the highway.

With the traffic spaced a quarter of a mile apart, I figured this was going to be a snap. Yet, as I looked up the road I could see a gold colored, beautifully restored muscle car really hauling ass down the highway. My guess was the car was doing at least 100 mph. I started to get an uneasy feeling. Seeing it rapidly overtaking the car in front of him, I watched the driver of the hot rod snap his car to the left to avoid rear-ending the car that was doing the speed limit directly in front of him.

With growing interest I waited to see what the next move would be by this Mario Andretti wannabe and I suspected it wasn't going to be pretty. Suddenly the screech of tires and black puffs of smoke instantly told a whole new ugly story—the driver had just lost control of his car. I established that the odds still had to be a million to one that I was in danger...I mean really...it was a beautiful day with light traffic....

A millisecond later I lowered those odds to a thousand in one, then a hundred to one. By now the hot rod was off the highway and crossing the grassy center median at a very, very high rate of speed.

"No way!" the skeptical optimist in me still insisted as I recalculated new odds at ten to one as two tons of hardened steel started to bear down on my sweet behind. "Way!" said the more seasoned pessimist in the back of my head.

For a brief moment, figuring one-to-one odds, I thought I could dodge to the left or right and avoid getting killed. Those hopes ended in a flash, as the car fishtailed and presented me its entire broadside at 50 mph. When that happened all hope of jumping out of the way was eliminated and I came to that frightening, inexorable conclusion... "Oh God, I'm dead!"

WHAM! I remember the tremendous thudding sound of impact as my body caved in that old Ford Fairlane's front fender. It was an unpleasant sound, considering that my body was the source of it. Suddenly I was on a wild ride into a blinding white light while looking down and seeing myself lying in a ditch about a rooftop's distance below. My first thought was, "Dad, I never thought I'd beat you to this place. And Dad, after all our theological discussions and philosophical musings, I'm here to tell you that death, like we had always thought, is a conscious state."

It felt great to be dead, still able to think but no longer constrained by my physical being. I watched people touching me down in the ditch. I felt exhilarated and ready to move on. "Okay God, what's next?" was my most sublime acceptance of the hereafter. I was really enjoying myself.

Then the thought came to me, "What about Peggy and the kids???" Then I figured "Heh, they'll be with me in the blink of an eye.... Boy, this is great!" I felt spectacularly unencumbered and free. In an instant, I fully comprehended and accepted the meaninglessness of TIME. It was an antiquated idea created by mere earthbound mortals—a totally unique human contrivance invented solely to measure worth and accomplishment. It held no meaning at all to any other forms of life on earth, not to animals, not to plants, and, as I looked down at my body in the ditch, certainly not to newly dead people. Time had no meaning or relevance whatsoever. During this "state of lightness" or whatever the hell you want to call it, I felt my mind and spirit advance out beyond the stars. In the big picture, I mean the really big picture, time, space, distance, structure, weight, dimension—these things have no meaning—only spirit does.

It was at this point that I remember the voices getting louder and a woman screaming. I remember saying to myself, "Heh, you may not be dead after all." But this came as a surprisingly disappointing realization as I concluded that if I was alive, I surely must be paralyzed from a broken neck or back.

"Wiggle your hands, wiggle your toes," I commanded when I realized I was no longer looking down on myself and surmised I must be back "home" inside my body. With feelings coming from my fingers and toes, I concluded that I was not only alive but I was not paralyzed. Realizing I was still alive saddened me because my momentary "out-of-body" experience had been the most spectacular and profound adventure I'd ever experienced. I hungered for more. I had been ready.

Now I knew I'd have to function and live once again within all the limitations and ground rules placed upon those of us living in a physical and a material world.

I then started to feel heart-wrenching guilt for my utter willingness to abandon Peggy and our children. I hadn't asked to come back, it just happened. No matter how much I tried to rationalize that they would be with me "in the blink on an eye" I felt remorse for my willingness to leave them. What kind of husband and father was I?

Now, fully aware that I was daydreaming in a muddy ditch, I remember peering through the grass upside down at a dark-haired guy standing in the distance in front of a great looking car with a caved in right fender. I guessed he must have been the driver of the car. As someone started to roll me over, a woman shrieked, "Don't move him! His back might be broken!"

I was starting to feel bad about causing all this commotion. As a member of the rescue squad strapped me onto a wooden stretcher to fully immobilize my body, I told him, "I'm a Navy pilot, take me to the Navy Hospital."

In the Navy hospital emergency room, I was sore all over the place, but it was my knee that was really hurting. It had swollen up to the size of a watermelon. The doctors determined that the right side of my body had caved in the heavy steel of the old Ford.

I remembered jumping up an instant before I was hit so that the car would not go over the top of me, but instead send me airborne, just like I had learned from years of playing football. If I had planted my feet or crouched down, I am absolutely convinced the collision would have killed me. The car would have run over the top of me instead of allowing me to log a couple seconds of flight time. That little leap of faith saved my life.

In the emergency room, I heard a State Trooper tell doctors an eyewitness saw me get struck by the Ford and do six cartwheels ten feet in the air. The trooper had measured from the point of impact to the ditch where I was found. I had flown over 45 feet through the air. Just another couple of feet and I could have made it from third base to home plate—or into the northbound lanes of traffic on I-295.

Convinced I had internal bleeding, a female surgeon came running into the emergency room with a long, clear, soft plastic hose. "Uh...what's that for?" I asked, already knowing the answer and totally dreading her response.

"It's an urethral catheter. Why do you ask?"

"Well...it's so...BIG!?! The diameter looked a tad extreme. "Can I try to stick it inside the tube instead of sticking the tube inside it?!?"

Well, I begged and pleaded and even offered a bribe, all to no avail. Let me tell you something, a guy hasn't lived life as a man until he's had an urethral catheter placed deep inside him without a sedative or muscle relaxant. What a test of manhood! What a rite of passage! Four times they rammed it in and three times they pulled it out while trying to get the three feet of tubing seated inside my bladder. UUUghh...I still shudder to think about it. On the fourth try, just as I was about to pass out from the pain, it seated. Once the catheter was in place, I passed blood-free urine, which was quite a disappointment to me after what I had just suffered.

I heard my friends from work—who had been called in by

the hospital—laughing hysterically in the hall outside the emergency room. They had been listening all along and had immensely enjoyed the whole experience—every inch of it. I needed some new friends. Previously, I had been nicknamed "Goshawk" by another Navy pilot, Ken Haizlip. Although this nickname stuck with me, my secretary took full advantage of my hospital bed bound existence and began to refer to me as "Commander Roadkill." She even presented me a framed letter of commendation. Stuck in the center of it under the glass was a piece of garbage from the box I had dragged off I-295. It stated, "Presented to 'Freeway Goss' for Being a Conspicuous Obstacle in the Line of a Car."

When I got the terrifying phone call that Bill had been struck by a car on Interstate 295, my first thought was that Bill had probably stopped to help a turtle or snake get across the road. He has never had the heart to knowingly leave small animals on a busy roadway to get run over. He has always had that much love and respect for life.

When I heard he had stopped to get a large box of garbage off the highway, I thought it was odd until I remembered seeing him drag tree limbs and large rocks off the road even though we had safely passed them. It all made sense to me then.

"But, he's going to be okay" quickly followed from the mouth of one of Bill's friends from work. Somehow, I already knew that. Bill had been knocked down but never out, and he would always rise again. The guy I married has nine lives...like a cat...a big cat...a jaguar. My problem was I didn't know what number he was on.

Four days after the accident, I convinced Catheter Woman, Batman's sidekick if he had been a urologist, to release me from the hospital. Beat up, but alive, I started the P-3 Orion Refresher Flight Training syllabus the next day. Soon I was flying again, and although I love to fly, I quickly realized that aviating big airplanes on long flights with a bum knee, a bad wrist, a sore back and a whole new perspective on life would be a challenge. I just didn't know how much challenge—or how much more self-motivation—still remained in me to continue pursuing a military aviation career.

Lying in bed one night I reflected on my "out-of-body" experience. Did I die from shock and then come back? Or was my body knocked so instantaneously and violently that the aura of my spirit and soul was temporarily displaced until they could find their way back to my body? Or was I just full of crap? These were perplexing questions for someone who always wanted to quickly achieve a solution to a problem and then move on.

I later reminded my father how, years earlier, he had emphatically told me to never drive past something in the road that might cause other people to have an accident. Quickly he rebutted, "But, Billy—I never thought you would do it!" Then he gave me a bearhug and laughed, amazed that his youngest son was still alive.

I completed the four-month refresher training with a performance that lacked my normal fire. I also completed my Department Head tour at Patrol Squadron Forty-Five in a similar fashion. One of the high points of the refresher training was a week of flying in and out of Holland. I had another aviation article published in *Approach*, the technical magazine read by military aviators. This article concerned a complete loss of navigational equipment at nighttime in the middle of the North Atlantic. It occurred while I was the senior pilot on an operational flight from France to Iceland. Not a good predicament to be in.

This story will help to illustrate the complexities of piloting sophisticated military aircraft. It also clarifies how important it is to have both management and analytical skills—as well as the prerequisite requirement of good hand/eye coordination—

to pursue a Navy flying career. Finally this condensed article makes clear something especially true in aviation—that some days you're lucky and some days you're not—but usually it's a combination of both.

DEAD RECKONING NAVIGATION:
KNOCK THE RUST OFF
By Lt. Cmdr. Bill Goss, U.S. Navy

Our antisubmarine warfare crew had just completed a three-day detachment to France. We were flying home at 24,000 feet, on top of a heavy overcast layer of clouds talking on the radios to Oceanic Radio. Around 450 miles south of our island destination, Keflavik, Iceland, the Copilot reported losing our #2 inertial (an inertial is a piece of electronic navigational equipment that uses gyroscopes for determining movement and changes in position). He turned the inertial off and switched the attitude source to the standby gyro. Our first inertial had already failed soon after we had taken off. Now we had none. Both electrically powered compasses began to move erratically. Then everything failed. We told the Navigator he now had to use our primitive wet compass as our primary source for navigating.

Since we had eight hours of fuel and the weather was reported good at Keflavik, I was not overly concerned. We could still navigate like in the old days by dead reckoning, using the wet compass and divert if necessary. However, I was still surprised by some of the events that followed, especially in an aircraft that normally has as much navigational capability as the P-3C Update III.

I started doing short counts on the VHF radio so that the Air Traffic Controller in Iceland could use a direction finder to tell us what bearing we were from him. We had tuned all available ADF frequencies, even a powerful rock and roll radio station suggested by the Controller to no avail. Finally, we got a good point on the Keflavik non-directional beacon. Moments later, the Controller reported a good bearing line off his direction finder and recommended a new heading change. Both indicated a 90-degree heading change to the right. We turned to this heading and a little while later were reported in radar contact at 162 miles from Iceland. We continued to the field and flew a radar-guided approach to an uneventful landing.

What did we learn? Sometimes we get over-confident with the sophisticated navigational capabilities of our airplanes and crews. Our simplest systems sometimes prove to be the best.

Dead Reckoning navigation in a P-3C might not be as remote a possibility as you think. Train for it. If you start dead reckoning, do not forget (or confuse) the mnemonic device "Can Dead Men Vote Twice at Elections?" to remember the rule "Compass Deviation Magnetic Variation True Add East."

The Navigator made the "simple" error of subtracting 20 degrees west variation instead of adding it to develop a recommended magnetic heading. Also, the Navigator did not keep an off-line navigation log, thus restricting the Tactical Coordinator's ability to check the Navigator's computations. Ultimately, this provided the flight station with a course of 319 degrees instead of 359 degrees magnetic, an extremely significant 40 degree heading error.

I'd say it's time to knock the rust off our DR Navigation equipment and start training on it like your life depended on it—it just may!

If we had stayed on the course that the Navigator had figured for us we would have missed Iceland by a couple of hundred miles. We would have run out of gas late that night, being forced to make a gear up landing on the ice somewhere south of the North Pole. I learned a lot that night. If we had been lucky—very lucky—we would have spent the night in an igloo. But somehow, I didn't think so.

As much as I hated being separated from my family for months at a time, I still enjoyed the camaraderie and esprit de corp that exists among military people on deployment. They all hated being away from home as much as the next person. The best were able to compartmentalize those feelings and work through them. Initially I had the ability to compartmentalize my feelings to a fine science. But this ability diminished somewhat after the children were born. And, after the "out-of-body" experience, I seemed to lose the knack for compartmentalizing almost entirely. But I continued to enjoy the relationships with other members of the squadron and tried hard to use humor to help raise others' spirits when they were feeling down.

I particularly enjoyed my relationship with other officers in the wardroom. Historically, there is always a friendly rivalry between the fifty or so Lieutenants and Lieutenant junior grades and the six to eight Lieutenant Commanders in the squadron. The junior officers (JOs) were members of JOPA which stood for the Junior Officer Protection Association. The junior officers referred to the senior pilots and senior naval flight officers as being members of SORA, the Senior Officer Retirement Association. This friendly rivalry was an important element of the esprit de corp of the squadron and was generally condoned by the executive and commanding officers.

The SORA in our squadron formed a secret society within the squadron. That really confused JOPA. We called ourselves the BOBS, which in our "code" was the self-deprecating acronym for the Big Old Butts. Compared to 25-year-old lieutenants, our butts were bigger and older. I was dubbed BOB SENIOR, having been blessed with the oldest and biggest butt of the group, unlike the bony little butts of the younger junior officers. In close order, the "BOBS" were Greg Miller as BOB JUNIOR, Bill Moran as BILLY BOB, Pat "Bo" Mills as BO BOB, Tim "Pink" Floyd as PINK BOB, Phil "Mo" Farrell as MO BOB, and Bill "Claw" Cloughley as CLAW BOB. The Wing Commander we worked under was named Bob, our Commanding Officer's name was Bob, and our Executive Officer's name was Rob. So, if you are following any of this, we called ourselves "Bob and Bob and Rob's BOBS."

When members of JOPA drank at the Brass Nut, our tiny squadron officers' club in Iceland, they would get obnoxious and attempt to bug us because it was part of their charter as members of JOPA to annoy the Department Heads. We would commence with our Bob talk and start their heads reeling. It would sound something like this:

"Heh, Senior, you seen any of the BOBS around?"

"No, Junior, which BOB you talking 'bout? Mo Bob, Bo Bob, Billy Bob, Pink Bob, or Claw Bob?"

"Neither. Senior, your Bob's shrinking. You working out?"

"Yeah, a little, but I sure don't want that to happen!"

"Hell no, Senior! What do you think about us BOBS getting our bobs back up to size by eating some of those cookies the Bobettes sent up here?"

We parted utilizing our infamous BOB goodbye. "Junior...Senior...As always...."

By this time, the Junior Officers sitting near us at the bar would get up and move elsewhere, completely disgusted that they couldn't comprehend a conversation that they hoped would hold some meaningful dirt on one of the other JOs. It was some of the most meaningless, and yet meaningful, repartee of the deployment. Steeped in humor it helped quell the loneliness we all felt being so far from home and from our wives and children. I even found a "bible" for our group, an outrageously funny book titled *Three-Fisted Tales of "BOB."* Bob Junior would keep it at his desk where we would all refer to it daily to keep up our spirits.

The BOBS referred to my car accident as an example of "...when Senior went BOBBING IN A NO BOB ZONE..."

Although the department head tour is a relatively short period of time, we BOBS have continued to stay much "tighter" than most Department Heads ever did. As Bob Junior was forever fond of saying, "Senior, we're too much—aren't we?"

After the Iceland deployment, I realized I could no longer put my family and myself through any more extended separations. It was just too tough on all of us. While in the Navy, I had been on ten deployments out of the country for periods lasting from two to eight months, with most lasting six. I started to realize my family life and my married life could only be stretched so thin. If I really loved my family, I had to find a way to spend more time with them. And I wanted to decide "to where and how long" I'd be away and not have that decision made for me by some higher authority or dictated by circumstance. My family could handle me being away for six days—but no longer for six months.

After the car accident and his bizarre out-of-body experience, I detected a change in Bill. He became more of a family man and less of a Navy man. He was more introspective and less extroverted. I knew that this accident had put his career in an uncompromising position. Naturally for Bill, he started Flight Refresher Training on crutches just a day or two after being released from the hospital. But, I noticed a lot of his natural competitiveness had left him and he no longer cared about the semi-annual rankings of the officers. Having always strived to be ranked number one, Bill wasn't the same. He no longer felt the need to prove himself to the world. I thought it was nice to see this change in him but a bit scary, too. I wondered, "What was to become of him?"

I requested a transfer to the Admiral's staff and it was approved. Peg and I were delighted. It meant we could stay in our home by the St. John's River on historic Fleming Island, and finally give the kids a place to call home.

Admiral Dirren and his wife, Susan, were wonderful people and consequently it was a pleasure to work for him. I represented the Admiral in a myriad of interesting duties. One of these assignments was to be one of three jury members on one of the very last Tailhook trials. Called a Board of Inquiry, our three member jury had the power to terminate the career of the Lieutenant who sat before us, a young jet pilot accused of "reaching toward" a woman while a part of the infamous Tailhook "gauntlet."

It was a compelling case but there was no evidence against the accused and no witnesses spoke against him. An investigation team from the DOD found another pilot who stated that he had allegedly seen the Lieutenant reach out in an attempt to touch someone, but this same witness eventually retracted his statement against the accused by claiming he had been fatigued into making his earlier statement.

Ultimately, the entire case had been built on a tiny amount of hearsay, which was later withdrawn. The three of us on the jury—one female Supply Corps Commander and two Naval Aviator Lieutenant Commanders—deliberated for only a few minutes before coming out with a not guilty verdict on all three counts. Even though there was absolutely no evidence at all that could have possibly led to a conviction, this young Navy pilot suffered as a scapegoat for years while more senior personnel looked the other way.

The Tailhook Convention at the Las Vegas Hilton had been a setting for disgraceful behavior for many years. Free flowing alcohol, no uniforms and no accountability could not possibly lend itself towards enhanced professionalism. I don't know how anybody ever thought it could. I learned as a member of that jury that no matter how screwed up Tailhook was the investigations that followed were worse. Many of them appeared to be witch-hunts moving forward with little or no meaningful evidence. And the injustice of it all was that the most junior officers seemed to suffer the most, even though similar Tailhook conventions had been condoned for years by very senior people in the Department of Defense. Slapstick is one thing, but physically and verbally abusing women is something entirely different. It is supposed to be an "officer and a gentlemen" not an "officer or a gentlemen."

Finally, while working for the Admiral, I had the opportunity to fly the new Lamps MK60 helicopter simulator. Its simulation of landing on ships at sea was the ultimate in virtual reality. I also got to fly the two seat version of the supersonic FA-18 Hornet with Captain Bruce Hilgartner of the U.S. Marine Corps, a close friend and fighter pilot at a nearby squadron. Going supersonic and breaking the sound barrier off the coast of Florida was the apex of my flying career. What a wild ride it was!

It was also my last flight as a U.S. Navy Pilot.

CHAPTER NINE

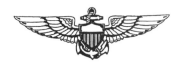

WHAM!
GOSS COLLIDES WITH CANCER

*"What lies behind us and what lies before us, is nothing
compared to what lies within us."*
—Emerson

S hortly after the awesome experience of breaking the
sound barrier in the FA-18 Hornet, I found a small clear
skin bump on the back of my left ear. When I mentioned to a
group of friends that I had this pea-size bump behind my ear
everyone else responded, "Oh, you do—so do I." But when my
mother saw that bump, she told me I should have a doctor to
take a quick look at it. Mothers know stuff about their kids
that is sometimes simply unexplainable—even to them.

Taking my mother's advice, I went to the doctor only to be
told it was nothing to worry about. It was simply a harmless
fatty cyst that would go away on its own in a few months. It
took quite a bit of persuasion that day to get the doctor to remove it, but she did. Thankfully, without my knowing it, she
sent it to the Navy Hospital Pathologist, Dr. Elie, for evaluation.

Dr. Elie's report stated the "cyst" was instead a "tumor"
and "highly suspicious of malignant melanoma"—in other
words, cancer. Later, I sought him out in the hospital laboratory and he showed me some smashed cells from my left ear
under his high powered microscope. He made a point of show-

ing me how my biopsy was full of misshapen cells with numerous nuclei in each cell, typical of malignant cancer. He explained how melanoma cells accept various stains differently than other cancers and so he'd sent some of my tumor to the Armed Forces Institute of Pathology (known as the AFIP in medical lingo) for a very specific type of staining technique and a much more conclusive diagnosis.

I knew cancer wasn't good news, but I was just ignorant enough to believe that cancer from this tiny bump behind my ear couldn't be too bad. I mean—really—it was just a little bump. After all, I felt pretty good, still able to go to work. I still had some aches and pains from when I got run down by the Ford, but that was to be expected. I pushed hard to have the required surgery done immediately to stop it from spreading and to start the healing process right away. Of course, I didn't think the surgery would be a big deal, just a slightly deeper cut on the ear. Lord, how wrong I was.

I was referred immediately to Navy Surgeon Lieutenant Commander Bob Fisher at the hospital's ENT (Ears, Nose and Throat) clinic. Doc Fisher gave me devastating news. Due to the location and the very significant depth of the tumor, my prognosis was very poor. I had asked him to be direct and honest with me, and he was. "You could be dead in six months." From the look in his downcast eyes, I could tell he didn't believe I could be dead in six months; he believed I would be dead in six months.

It's hard to explain what it's like when one day you've never given the word "cancer" a moment's thought, and the next day you feel that thinking about that same word will consume every moment and every second of the rest of your life. But, that is exactly what happens when you hear the three most dreaded words in the English language—"You've got cancer."

He further explained that the biopsy removed had a lack of connective cancer cells to the skin cells, which meant that the tumor in my ear had a high probability of being a metastatic deposit from an unlocated primary tumor, hidden somewhere else in my body.

Terminal cancer? Me? No way! I was in a state of shock. First getting hit by the out-of-control car and now this. This couldn't be happening to me.

My parents urged me to get a second opinion from a civilian doctor before I agreed to any surgery. It sounded like good advice to me. "Besides," I thought, "these Navy doctors must simply be mistaken. Suspicious of cancer...maybe. Terminal...NEVER!"

The next day I talked with my longtime buddy, Billy Beal, who lived nearby. He asked a doctor friend of his to talk about my case with Dr. Cassisi, the head of the ENT Department at University of Florida's Shands Hospital in Gainesville. Weekly at Shands, Dr. Cassisi leads the Tumor Board, the purpose of which is to give the patient a multidisciplinary approach to treating their cancer. After talking to me on the phone, a concerned Dr. Cassisi arranged for me to be examined by the medical board members the next morning.

During the two-hour drive to Gainesville to be examined by the Tumor Board, I convinced myself that they would determine it was a tumor, but a benign one—simple to remove and treat. "No way could this happen to me!" I rationalized to myself. "I've lived too healthy a life. Cancer is for people who don't look after themselves—smokers and drinkers and sungods and people who eat like disgusting pigs. And I've tried to look after myself pretty damn well—well, except for the eating, that is. Me with cancer...no way!"

Since Doc Fisher had given me such bad news already, I was prepared for the worst; but I still expected better than what I got. The Tumor Board concluded that I had a deep, deadly and very difficult to diagnose cancer of the melanocytes—the melanin producing skin cells—the same cells that darken your skin with a tan. Malignant melanoma typically begins as a somewhat normal looking mole that becomes uglier and darker looking as the skin cells that produce melanin suddenly begin to reproduce at an out-of-control rate.

My melanoma tumor had been so difficult to diagnose because it was without any melanin or dark pigmentation, medically termed as being "amelanotic." My little bump was not ugly or black but smooth and clear like regular skin. In other words, it was easy to ignore. Due to the insidious nature of this form of cancer, it is so deadly because by the time it normally causes people—or doctors—to take it seriously, it will have spread to major organs in the person's body. According to researchers, amelanotic melanoma only shows up at the secondary sites, not at the primary tumor.

Finally, one of the doctors at the Tumor Board told me I should "get my estate in order." I couldn't believe it. I was only 38-years-old! He had discovered a swollen lymph node in my neck, near my left jugular vein, six inches below the tumor in my ear. This was really bad news, terrifying news. I pretended that the blinding white examination light was making my eyes water and asked them to turn it away from my face.

A renowned surgeon of vast experience, Dr. Cassisi advised even more radical surgery than Dr. Fisher had proposed. Along with the removal of some or all of my left ear, about 200 lymph nodes, the trapezius muscle and probably the jugular vein, he also wanted the large salivary gland, known as the Parotid, removed from under the left side of my face. I could expect facial paralysis and constant drooling to be some of the temporary and possibly permanent side effects.

One certainty was that I would endure a lot of pain and disfigurement as a result of the estimated eleven-hour operation. The operation wasn't going to be pretty—and neither was I going to be when they were done with me.

Radiation therapy would be necessary if any lymph nodes tested positive for cancer. A lymph node evaluated as positive for malignant cell growth would clearly establish that the tumor had spread into my lymphatic system. If a tumor is found at a more distant site than a nearby lymph node it may be indicative of metastatic disease—reputedly incurable for malignant melanoma. Called the "Tyrannosaurus Rex of Cancers" by newsman and fellow melanoma survivor Sam Donaldson, it is a terribly vicious malignancy.

After I left Shands Hospital, Dr. Cassisi discussed by phone his evaluation and recommendations with Dr. Fisher, who was still awaiting the pathology reports from the AFIP before he could schedule my surgery. I had been told earlier the AFIP had a very specific kind of cell staining procedure that would be able to prove once and for all that my tumor biopsy was indeed malignant melanoma. The waiting for the AFIP results was unmerciful. I was ready for the cutting to begin and I would have done it myself if I could have. I wanted this tumor out of my body and I wanted it out now. It felt like Peggy and I had to wait, and wait, and wait. God knows, I never knew a few weeks could last an eternity.

So here I was—terrified at the thought of leaving my wife and my children behind while they were still so young—trying to figure out what the hell to do next. The pea sized, clear-skin lump I had to insist be removed from the back of my left ear had earlier been diagnosed as a harmless cyst. Now it was trying to kill me. How I'd turn this into a positive learning experience was beyond me.

Some doctors have indicated to me that severe trauma, like when I was knocked 45 feet through the air by the out-of-control car, can have a profound negative effect upon a person's auto-immune system—no pun intended. It's as good a reason as any as to why my immune system allowed this tumor to develop. I tried to think of any other rational explanations as to why this would happen to me—but I just couldn't come up with anything.

While waiting for a thumbs up from the AFIP, I went to the library to research my disease and my life expectancy. The first step was to look up the definition of the word "malignant" in the dictionary. It read "Pathol. deadly; tending to produce death, as a disease or tumor." Next, I checked out the *Merck Manual of Diagnosis and Therapy*, the widely accepted bible of modern medicine now in its sixteenth edition. Under the headings of "Malignant Melanoma," I read the following:

> "...may spread so rapidly that it will be fatal within months of recognition. . . lymphocytic infiltration is maximal in the most superficial lesions, it decreases with the deeper levels of tumor cell invasion."

For cancers of Unknown Primary Origin:

> "These patients account for 0.5% to 7% of all cancer patients...survival in patients with cancers of an unknown primary origin is generally poor (median is 3-4 months)....Metastatic melanoma cannot be cured at present."

I quickly calculated that the 0.5% meant the odds were 200 to 1 against me. "Oh my God!" I cried out in a private corner of the library. Again I cried out, this time to Jesus, out to the heavens, "Christ, why me?"

"Why not?" was the simple reply that echoed back.

I wasn't afraid to die, but I was sick with grief at the thought of leaving my wife and children to find their way without me. I felt I had already abandoned them once when I was run down by the car and it was God's desire, not mine, that had me fall back to Earth. Why then would he want to come get me a few years later? Was this one more test of my character?

Early one morning, unable to sleep due to acute anxiety, I got up and went outside to take a leak under the immensity of the stars. Guys do that, sometimes. I stood, barefoot in the sweet smelling grass wet with the morning dew (and other things). Looking into the star-studded universe I asked, "God, if you are listening to my prayers, to my heart, please Lord, oh please...show me a sign." I waited, face pointed to the heavens. After a few minutes, with the task at hand complete and with an aching neck to boot, I said to myself "This is stupid—what am I waiting for?" I started to turn to go inside. At that moment the largest meteor I've ever seen, a blinding white fireball, went from the southern horizon clear across the sky to the North, like it was beckoning me to follow. Lasting a good five seconds, I collapsed onto the porch step and watched the golden streak of ionized air the giant meteor left behind slowly twinkle into oblivion.

Face in hands, I started to cry, one of the most gut-wrenching, soul shaking, most fearful and thankful cries of my life. For God to wait until the exact moment at which my shallow faith failed before lighting my way through this adversity was my just dessert. I no longer felt the anguish of feeling alone and separate from the universe for I now knew it was a part of me and I was part of it. It was like I had been lost forever in a darkened room when suddenly my fingers happened upon the light switch. Suddenly, I could see. With adversity comes "light" if you only look long enough for it. In fact, the light is always there.

I now knew that the Lord was listening to me and always had been. God is real, prayer is powerful, and faith, even small amounts, means everything.

With a powerfully renewed feeling of hope after seeing God's monster meteor, I set out to learn everything possible about malignant cancer from information sent to me by caring doctors and specialists I befriended across the country.

Immediately I started drinking a tea called Essiac formulated many moons ago by the Ojibway Indian tribe. It is made from burdock root, sheep sorrel, turkey rhubarb root, slippery elm bark and other secret herbs, all of which grow abundantly in North America. Many scientists are discovering that compounds such as inulin, contained within burdock root, can serve as powerful immune system modulators in human subjects. I was willing to explore every root—I mean route—to survival.

The tea was sent to me by Dr. Pierre Gaulin, a forensic pathologist and Mohawk/Abenaki Indian, from Canada. A holistic medicine man with impeccable credentials, Rat, who had lost his father to cancer, somehow hunted him down on the Internet and utilizing his remarkably persuasive skills, got Pierre to call me. This wonderful man took personal interest in me, a total stranger, through his many phone calls and faxes. He and his wife, Rose, even went out of their way to visit Peggy and me on their annual pilgrimage from Fort Lauderdale to Canada. As I led Dr. Gaulin, a handsome man in a three-piece suit, through my front door, I noticed he had a long thin pony tail trailing down his back. "This was no ordinary doctor," I said to myself. Pierre also told me to start taking odorless dried garlic twice a day, declaring it one of the most powerful life extending herbs on earth. I followed his Essiac and garlic orders to a tea—I mean tee.

Eighteen months later, I read that "researchers at University of California in L.A. discovered that aged garlic extract may prevent and control melanoma, a deadly skin cancer." Who could've figured? Certainly not me. And maybe Essiac and garlic have no positive effect on my health other than a placebo effect. Well, that's fine with me too. As long as it has some kind of positive effect on my attitude and mood then I believe my immune response is enhanced. But I do feel that Essiac and garlic does have an organic basis for helping my body fight disease. Just please don't ask me to try and explain it.

I was starting to see the good side of doctors, and I found that most have a very caring, very generous side. Old "home boy" friends, who "were never going to amount to anything" so they became doctors, such as Carl "The Gureenie" Guarino, "Big Al" Speidell and Scott Campbell, offered tremendous support through their nearly limitless expertise and resources. Even "Dr. Rat," the only practicing non-licensed physician I know, offered up his vast knowledge of biology and analytical chemistry to me. Without my faith, the love of my family and the support of friends, it would have been like being lost in the desert, something I was vaguely familiar with. Peggy's brothers and sisters helped out, searching the Internet and faxing me mountains of data on malignant melanoma. I wished I had this many friends when I was well.

Through my studies, I came to appreciate the fact that our

skin is our body's largest organ—not the lungs, heart, or brain. Nor any other organ despite what a lot of macho men would like to tell you. We've got to take damn good care of it. Many doctors believe that melanomas probably originate from a bad sunburn as a child and emerge as a malignancy years later. But, science has not established with absolute certainty the mechanics behind a good melanocyte going bad and becoming a tumor, at least not in a way that can be duplicated time and time again in a petri dish for control study purposes.

Anyhow, I used the light across the sky and the drinking of the Ojibway Indian tea to rebuild my mental fortitude. I developed the strength and resolve to fight this disease head on and even try to turn back the clock if the cancer had already microscopically infiltrated my lymphatic system. Late at night I would go out running, my right knee still aching from its encounter with the old Ford. While running I'd pray that my surgery date would come quickly, hoping the pain in my knee would help take away the pain in my heart—a heart which was breaking when I thought of Peggy and the twins. The three weeks of waiting for the go ahead from AFIP was torturing me.

When the Armed Forces Institute of Pathology completed their evaluation of my tumor slides with the special melanoma stain, they gave the go ahead to Dr. Fisher. It was now official.

The goal was to remove all possible traces of this deadly cell growth from the body of Lieutenant Commander Goss—me—immediately. I pleaded with them to start cutting. Every additional second that this malignancy remained in my body was one more second, one more opportunity, for it to spread—to my brain, my heart, my lungs, my stomach—you name the organ and melanoma can invade it—with devastating results.

Being a very lengthy operation, mine had to be planned well ahead. Still Doc Fisher, along with some concerned phone calls from Admiral Dirren and his Chief of Staff Captain O'Neil, somehow managed to coordinate the surgery to commence at seven a.m. the next morning.

I remember saying to Doc Fisher before going under anesthesia:

"Doc, will I be able to play the piano when this is all over."

"Of course you will, Commander Goss."

"That's wonderful, Doc, because I could never play a lick before."

"Go to sleep, Bill," he chuckled.

All strapped in with no place to hide, I laid on that hospital gurney kissing Peggy goodbye. With our hands clenched together like we'd never let go, we waited for the sedative dripping into my left forearm to take hold. I knew I'd be a changed man when I awoke—I just didn't know how changed.

I gagged violently while desperately trying to puke. An alcohol smell filled my nose and the world was painted in a nauseating purple haze. I felt a hand on my forehead. "He's coming to." The nurse called to Peggy. The revolting veil of purple haze slowly lifted as a sterile blue-green hospital cloth was taken off my swollen eyes, suddenly blinding me with the bright megawatt lights of the intensive care unit. If I had never wanted to die before, I did now. I gagged again and choked on a large steel tube that had been rammed down my throat.

Prior to surgery, I had been told that the longer I was under general anesthesia the longer and more violently ill would be my recovery. "I must have been under for eons...." I thought as my head exploded, my heart raced and I tried to vomit again. My heavily stapled throat strained on the large steel endotracheal tube.

"Can you take that thing out of his throat?" Peggy gently asked the nurse as I squeezed her hand a thank you.

"Yeah, I think he's ready now," the nurse said as she pulled out what looked like a silver trowel.

I thought, "Oh, my God, I can't believe I ate the whole thing!" I had another bout with dry heaves at the thought of that giant metal thing coming out of my mouth. Struggling to help the nurses move me from the operating gurney to a bed, I placed my hands at my side and tried to sit up. In that one unlucky movement, I inadvertently yanked on all the plastic tubes that had been planted deep in my face and neck wounds to suck out blood and lymph. They were irreplaceable and it proved to be a terrible stroke of misfortune.

A few hours later, as the blinding nausea began to ease up, the incredible pain began. I slowly felt my face and neck, my fingers not yet working in concert with my brain. I was mummified, wrapped in blood-soaked bandages. Then I became aware of the noise. I slowly moved my eyes to the left then to the right. I saw Peggy standing above me like an angel. I tried to talk to her to ask her what that hellacious sucking sound was, but my vocal chords had just had the living daylights beat out of them by that steel thing from hell. I just ugh, ugh, ughed her to death.

"Don't try to talk, Honey," she whispered. Again the awful sucking sound occurred like the flushing of an enormous toilet bowl. I saw her eyes widen. Then I knew that horrible sucking sound was coming from me. Earlier, when I had accidently pulled on the tubes in my wounds, I had unseated them and disrupted their vacuum and ability to successfully suck out the unwanted stagnating blood. Now instead the tubes were sucking mostly air. Without the blood and the clear, yellow lymph fluid being removed from my wounds, my face and neck had already swollen to gargantuan proportions.

I groaned from the pain. Another nurse, Lt. Jenny Candy, came over. "Can you understand me, Commander Goss?" she slowly asked, resting her hand on my forearm. I moved my eyeballs slowly up and down. "I'm going to hand you a little button. If you have pain, press this button and a small dose of morphine will drop into your veins. It's run by a little computer and automatically stops dosing when you've had enough. You can't overdose using it, understand?" Boy, did I ever. Click, Click, Click, in a few moments things weren't so bad after all.

In the days that followed I really became a "swell guy." The good doctors and Nurse Carol Otis took turns manually massaging and sucking the blood and lymphatic fluid from my neck with a gigantic hypodermic needle to reduce the swelling. It was extremely unpleasant but absolutely necessary to prevent the blood from pooling and stagnating. Suddenly, fighting cancer was no longer the immediate concern. Fighting infections and reducing high fevers were now the critical element in my survival.

The third day after surgery was Peggy's and my fourteenth wedding anniversary. Finally, alone for a little while, I summoned up the strength to crawl out of bed to pretty myself for when Peggy arrived. When I finally saw myself in the mirror I nearly fainted. My blood covered pressure wrappings were almost black and the little bit of my face that was visible was swollen to twice its size. My face and eyes had the look of an obese man that a heavyweight prize-fighter had just beaten the living daylights out of. "You is one ugleee dude," I concluded while half laughing, half crying. I was also fervently praying that I'd be around one year later to celebrate our fifteenth anniversary and not look like Frankenstein.

Sleeping in the hospital was impossible. Just when I'd start to doze, the loudest, the most disgusting noise imaginable would rattle through my face and neck, sounding like a giant preschooler sucking up his runny nose. I begged the doctors to take me off the vacu-suck and send me home for some sleep. They finally did.

When I got home from the hospital, I still had a wrapping around my face and neck. Brian and Christie were shocked at my appearance at first. I explained to them how I was wrapped like a mummy. Christie loved the story and started calling me "Mummy Daddy."

While recovering at home, Peg and I had another very important waiting game called "Waiting for the Post-operative Pathology Report." Once again, this agonizing ordeal stretched unmercifully into almost two weeks. We waited to hear from the AFIP as to whether any of the approximately 200 lymph nodes taken from my face, neck, and ear were positive for melanoma.

It was the cancer that really took me by surprise. It was hard for me to understand how such a little bump behind Bill's left ear could be so serious. Waiting to see him after the eleven hours of surgery seemed to take an eternity. But, when I saw what he looked like when he came out of the operating room, I began to fully comprehend just how deadly this cancer must be. He had been torn to pieces and literally stapled back together. I wanted to cry. And where was his left ear? The whole top half was missing!

Suddenly, I realized that doctors wouldn't have done this to Bill unless he was seriously—very seriously—ill. We had previously agreed to be as honest as possible with Brian and Christie, who were age six at the time, without scaring or causing them nightmares. I quickly saw this wasn't going to be easy. Thank God they hadn't seen the movie Frankenstein.

"Illness is the doctor to whom we pay most heed: to kindness and to knowledge we make promises only—pain we obey."
—Marcel Proust

One thing all the post-operative pain taught me was how unappreciative I had become not having had significant amounts of pain in my past. Dr. Paul Brand, a missionary physician who wrote a book about pain titled *The Gift Nobody Wants*, argues that America's pursuit of pleasure and attempts at eliminating pain at all costs has actually had the opposite effect. He claims a double irony is at work. In conquering pain and not suffering we've inadvertently become less able to tolerate it. And, by endlessly seeking pleasure, we've created ever-rising expectations that keep true contentment just out of reach. The 80-year-old Dr. Brand says patients in the United States live "at a greater comfort level than any I had previously treated, but they seemed far less equipped to handle suffering and far more traumatized by it."

Understanding Dr. Brand's view of "pain and pleasure" not

as opposites, but as joined partners, was a thought-provoking new way to look at how I viewed human suffering. In my case the extreme pain of my surgery gave me unusual pleasure. It meant I had finally done what I prayed would be all I needed to rid my body of cancer.

I was weaned off morphine and put on codeine, another very powerful narcotic that affected me in wildly hallucinogenic ways. One night, I awoke completely convinced that I was dying of AIDS in the jungles of Vietnam. I woke Peggy to apologize to her. As she patiently rubbed her eyes at 3 a.m., I said, "Peggy, I'm so sorry. I have no idea how I got AIDS...I've never cheated on you, never, and now I'm gonna die!" That morning Peggy took me to Doctor Jeff Sandler's office for my routine blood letting ritual, putting a tap in my swollen throat like so many Tutzi tribesmen do to their goats.

As Peggy explained to Jeff how I hadn't been sleeping very well, I tried to interrupt. "Doc, could I go to the lavatory first?"

"Naw, Bill, this will only take a minute." He whipped out this enormous needle and plunged it into my neck. Well according to Peggy, as soon as he pulled blood from my neck, my blood pressure dropped and I passed out, falling over backwards, swallowing my tongue, and peeing in my pants. All three of those things were firsts for me. After Doc Sandler helped me regain consciousness, in a fog I once again asked him, "Doc, can I go to the bathroom now?"

He looked at my pants and politely responded, "Commander Goss, I think that's no longer necessary."

About this time, my brother Larry flew down from Rhode Island to cheer me up and to give Peggy a break from caregiving. He got a big laugh out of watching me try to put on sunglasses for the first time. They kept falling off my face because there was no left ear to hold them in place. "You're a real pathetic piece of work," Larry bemusedly exclaimed. The next day, he took me to the Navy hospital for a follow-up visit. While there, Doc Fisher came in with a computer printout in his hand. "Bill, your post-operative pathology report just came in from the AFIP."

"Yes?" I said, responding to his pregnant pause.

"Well, they reported that all your lymph nodes are grossly benign."

"What's so gross about them? Is that good news?"

"It sure is!"

"Time for a beer," Brother Larry stated factually.

After I told Peg the great news, Larry had me out on the St. John's River with my Navy buddies, Bo Mills and Frank Gren, eating hot chicken wings and drinking Coors. I'm sure the waitress was intimidated by the way I looked, having a partially paralyzed face with half an ear missing and big copper staples running up and down my neck. But she kept her sense of humor.

After the wonderful pathology report stating that none of my lymph nodes were positive for cancer (which would have spelled catastrophe with a capital "C"), I asked myself aloud, "What now?"

"Why don't you buy a sports car—a Porsche? You've never had one before," Brother Larry retorted enthusiastically. With the help of Mac McGehee, who not only looked at used Porsches for me but also volunteered some of his family fortune if necessary to ensure my survival, I ended up buying a gorgeous slate grey Porsche that was a trade-in at a nearby new car dealership. Ten years old, they were asking $8000 for it, but they sold it to me for $5000. Let me tell you, right after disfiguring surgery is a great time to bargain for a used car. Boy, do they ever want to get your ugly mug off the showroom floor!

What fascinated, amazed and amused my friends most of all was that I now drooled from a hole behind where my left ear once resided. It was truly disgusting—but what was I to do—go into isolation? I was never one to let a little spit ruin a good party.

After Doc Fisher removed my left parotid, our largest salivary gland, he had warned me about the possibly permanent side affects like facial paralysis and uncontrollable drooling and sweating in the presence of food. He told me that until the fistula behind my eardrum healed, I'd just have to live with the rain of spit emerging from it. Also, because saliva is composed mostly of digestive enzymes specially evolved for dissolving meat, it could take several months to heal.

First, it would squirt out from behind my ear. The saliva would then run down the side of my face and cascade from my chin to my lap. The tastier the food, the more torrential was the downpour. After a great meal, I'd carry a hat over the crotch of my pants as I left the restaurant because it would have soaked through all the napkins I had on my lap. Although I was concerned that people would think the big wet spot on the front of my pants was pee—the truth was even grosser—it was spit!

It wasn't long after my operation that I was notified that due to the severity of my condition and to the poor long-term prognosis for deep melanoma tumors—especially on the head—I would be medically retired for a service connected disability.

I was saddened to receive my retirement notification. It was tangible evidence that the organized and planned existence of my prior life had come to a loud screeching halt. But after 21 years in the U.S. Navy, with the last fifteen as a commissioned U.S. Naval Officer, my time had come. I will always be grateful for the opportunity I had to serve this great country of ours, both as an underwater explosives specialist and as a naval aviator. It had been one great adventure after another. Overall, it was an incredible experience—the memories of which I will forever cherish.

But I was also relieved. It was time to settle down and concentrate on one thing—my complete and total recovery. My goal now was to not only survive cancer, but to thrive in spite of it. And that was absolutely what I intended to do.

CHAPTER TEN

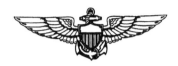

THE ROAD TO RECOVERY

"**H**ello, Commander Van Goss, please?" I recognized the voice immediately as Boobus. Now, Executive Vice President of Panavision Films in L.A., he was enjoying the good life with a house in Malibu and a wonderful job that took him all over the world. He had lost his mother to cancer when we were in college and was dumbstruck when I had told him about the cancer crisis I was dealing with.

"Well, Vincent, I guess you'll be getting your deposit money back for that five-day whitewater rafting trip we had planned," Boobus retorted.

Before I knew I had cancer, Boobus had invited me on a five-day whitewater rafting trip down the Colorado River in Utah. Now it was just weeks away and after the operation I had been through he was certain I'd have to cancel.

"Nope, I'll be there, Boobus." I said, grimacing in pain, as my stitches strained to break open while talking on the phone.

"Goss, you're crazy—see you there!" he said hanging up.

A few weeks later, equipped with a lot of protective clothing to shelter me from the sun, I was blasting through enormous Stage IV and V rapids with Boobus; his younger brother Freebs; Grazzoo; Bobby Sherman; the CEO of Panavision, Bill Scott; and his son David.

It was a fantastic trip, though not necessarily ideal for someone who was supposed to avoid exposure to the sun. Rafting through God's country, the upper Grand Canyon, was an amazingly life affirming experience. When the freezing water didn't numb the pain as my scars stretched and contracted, the ice-cold beer certainly did.

I highly recommend planning a trip like this after major surgery to remind yourself and your friends that you have no intention of sitting back and waiting for "something" to happen. Instead, prove to yourself that you are alive, more alive than ever before. Or just do it to tick off your doctors. The doctors might insist "Now let's take it easy for awhile...maybe something like that in a year or so when the odds are more in your favor...." Screw it, just do it. In my case, whitewater rafting in God's country was exactly what I needed to avoid slipping into postoperative depression.

Later Bill told me he was still going to go whitewater rafting down the Colorado River with the team from Panavision, even though his wounds had barely healed and he still suffered paralysis in his face. I thought he was crazy. But what else was new? It seemed just like the kind of adventure that Bill would seek out to prove to himself that "...yes, I'm still alive...."

It was sometime around my thirty-ninth birthday when I discovered that the 200 lymph nodes removed during my surgery were negative for cancer. I had been praying for two things and that was one of them. The other thing I prayed for was that my children never be stricken with a disease like this. The way I add extra umphf!!! to this prayer is that on the eve of my birthday—every birthday—I sit down and write a nice check to St. Jude Children's Research Hospital in Memphis, Tennessee. This remarkable medical center was founded by actor/comedian Danny Thomas and specializes in the treatment and curing of childhood cancers. Children who go there with cancer receive the finest and most compassionate medical treatment in the world. And it's all free as long as generous donations continue. I figured if there was a way to pray with your wallet—and I don't think there are many—this was it!

Let me tell you something—Mr. Spock had nothing over my left ear. Rising to a sharp point like a pencil eraser, it was impossible for people not to stare. Looking at it in the mirror, it would remind me of ten years ago when I went to my first—and last—bullfight in the Azores. After this particular bull was put to death, the matador proudly walked across the arena and looked me directly in the eyes. Then, with a quick snap of his wrist—like he was throwing a frisbee—the matador tossed me the bull's ear, still convulsing, right into my hands. The age-old tradition of the victorious matador was to toss an ear to the audience. Good fortune could be expected to visit upon the lucky person who caught the ear. And, if you placed that warm, bloody ear on a tavern bar later that night, you'd drink for free. What the hell, I figured. My father had always said, "When in Rome, do as the Romans do...."

Amazed at my catch, I gave a surprised nod of thanks to the matador as he gave me a pleased but unsettling look of providence that I had caught it. Later, after my friends and I had milked that ear for all it was worth at an Azorean tavern, I sat, watching Scooter ecstatically nibbling away on that big, black, hairy thing. I pondered what other uses for it I might dream up. I wondered then what stroke of good fortune the matador might have conjured up for me. Well, even though it was ten years too soon, it all made sense to me now. I finally understood what the matador was trying to convey to me with his thoughtful, sagacious look. It was "Here's an ear, buddy, cuz you're gonna need one!"

As the ear drooling problem slowed from a cascade to an occasional drip, and the deep indentations from the big metal staples started to fade, I began to look toward the future—not necessarily as a male model, but hopefully not as someone whose appearance would cause others to blow lunch. Half my face still suffered from paralysis, but it was slowly improving with the twice daily electrical stimulations the physical therapist had me doing. With one electrode glued below my eye and the other glued to my chin, I was encouraged to turn up the voltage as high as I could stand it. It was exactly how they jump-started Frankenstein, a shocking experience, to say the least.

Still fanatically studying about my disease, I learned that melanoma responds poorly to radiation treatments, and not at all to chemotherapy. It kills about 9000 Americans a year, many of them struck down in the prime of their life. Radiation can help buy a little time but it is so toxic that usually one full dose of radiation therapy is all one's body can take. In my case, the doctors felt that radiation should not be used unless a lymph node was found to be positive for melanoma tumor. This way, my natural immune system would not be fried and the one-shot radiation therapy could be saved until there was a need "to bring in the big gun."

At the time, the Navy hospital did not have a plastic surgeon on staff and the ENT surgeons would not consider doing ear reconstruction on me until one year had transpired from the date of the primary surgery. I had to wait out the period of time in which the cancer had its highest probability of recurring. To paraphrase one of the surgeons, "If we do an ear job on you and another tumor pops up, we'll have to radiate the whole mess, which will kill the new ear tissue and leave you with much less ear than before. Plus you'd be a goner anyway so it would just be a big waste of time."

I had asked my doctors not to pull any punches—to give me the straight, honest truth—and, once again, they had respected my wishes.

So, I waited as patiently as possible until my cancer-free one year anniversary finally arrived—eager to earn the privilege for plastic surgery to make right again my left ear.

Before I was able to have reconstructive surgery the pointed ear thing really started to bother me. I called a prosthetics company nearby to ask them if they had ever made a fake ear. "No" they said, "We've made lots of fake stuff, but no ears. We'd love to give it a try!" I figured with that kind of "Have silicone, will travel" attitude, I'd have to pay them a visit.

After making a plaster cast of my good ear and calling the "silicone guy" in Tampa, who specialized in making ears, noses, fingers, and probably glass fish tanks during his off months, I was quoted a price. "I didn't think an ounce of silicone could cost that much. Could we buy it in bulk quantities?" Not amused, I went to the Navy hospital to plead my case for the rubber ear. With a little ear pulling from the Admiral, they generously went along with it, being that it was a self-esteem thing and all.

A few weeks later, the prosthetist handed me a tube of glue, "Don't leave home without it," she dryly commented. Then out came this white thing from a box. "Here you go," the prosthetist exhorted as she glued it on.

"It's kind of white," I mumbled to myself, fascinated, as I looked at it in the mirror thinking it looked like a sleeping albino bat. Finally, unable to enjoy the folly any longer, I tugged till the Duco cement gave out and it popped off with a snap. "Can you send it back to the paint shed?" I asked. "Dutch Boy has a semi-gloss latex that's washable and available in Caucasian, and both African and Native American," I said smiling.

A week later, the new and improved ear arrived. The color was still off, though not nearly as bad as before. But the texture—well let's just say that silicone looks a whole lot better under the skin than on top of it. The prosthetics people had been wonderfully patient with me, as it was becoming very apparent that I didn't want a fake ear, I wanted my old one back.

After Duco cementing this one on, they sent me off to Dillard's Department Store to buy some cosmetics "to blend the whole thing together." At Dillard's, I tried to discreetly tell the cosmetics lady what I was trying to do. "Hey, Rita, come over here and help me with this guy's fake ear," she yelled across the counter to the other cosmetologist. Before long, I was sitting at the counter, arms and legs crossed just tittering away with these four nice ladies as we shared gossip and they put layer upon layer of blended goops on my ear in the hopes of giving it "that natural, just woke up look." After about an hour of being the store's featured ear cosmetics model and being nominated for the Orange Park Mall's "Spectacle of the Year" award, I figured it was time to depart the pattern (more aviator talk). As I stepped off the chair, I felt overcome by the weight on the side of my head from all the make-up that had been affixed to my ear and side of my face. And all this time I had thought it was bad backs that caused older women to walk hunched forward!

When I got home that afternoon, Peggy gasped as I walked through the door. In one swift movement, she yanked that little puppy from the side of my head, slid open my top dresser drawer and tossed it in. And that's where my fake ear has remained to this day, right next to the tube of Duco cement.

A brand-new kind of mouse that grew a human ear out of its back could have helped me out the most. Research scientists at the University of Massachusetts have almost miraculously found a way to make human cartilage cells grow into an ear-like shape while implanted under the skin on the back of a mouse. Specially designed and grown to manufacture faux human parts for use in plastic surgery, this mouse was biogenetically engineered to lack an immune system that rejects human tissue.

After the parasitic human ear has grown to its full size, it is removed from the mouse's back. Possibly it will be used on a toddler who was a victim of a dog bite or on a baby born without an ear. Unfortunately the genetically engineered mouse I refer to had grown a right ear—but I imagine a left-eared mouse will be on the drawing board real soon.

A year after Bill's recovery from his first surgery, our adorable little dog, Scooter, died of heart failure at age thirteen. This tore at our very souls. All four of us stroked her soft tiny inanimate body and wrapped her in one of Christie's favorite pink baby blankets. Broken-hearted, we sadly buried her in a shoebox under a tree by our pond. Christie put on the gravestone "Scooter...the best dog there ever was!"

Scooter's death was particularly sad for Bill and me. We had always thought of Scooter somewhat like our oldest child. For many years, there were just the three of us before our children were born. Scooter was incredibly lovable. She would always eagerly greet Bill at the door when he returned home and cover him with kisses as he lay down on the floor to return the sentiments. And during all those flying assignments and deployments, Scooter was my only companion. There were over a thousand days when Bill was gone and it was just "Scooter and me against the world." Scooter had helped both Bill and me get through many hard times.

Scooter's death was overwhelming for me. I knew she was older and she had developed some health problems. But mourning her death led me to reflect upon Bill's health and his life threatening experiences. Soon my overwhelming devastation was changed into a peaceful resolve. I realized that just as Scooter's life had been so purposeful to our family, so was her death. Scooter's passing had helped all of us remember and experience the temporal nature of life on earth. I remain thankful that it was only Scooter's life we needed to mourn, not Bill's.

As my inevitable medical retirement moved closer, so did my "Roadkill" litigation. At the trial, an accident reconstruction engineer stated, and I'm paraphrasing, "After calculating the weight of the victim with the distance he traveled through the air after impact, in conjunction with depth of the dents in the heavy steel of the offending 1965 Ford Fairlane, the force of impact upon Lt. Commander Bill Goss's body was the equivalent of him having stepped off a ten story building and landing on a cement driveway." He then showed the jury the police report that stated my measured takeoff to landing distance was 45 feet. My lawyer then passed around photographs of the damaged car and shots of the takeoff and landing zones as evidence.

The insurance company's lawyer argued that it wasn't his client's fault—even though his client had already paid an uncontested fine for careless driving. The lawyer instead placed the blame on the car in front of his client that "obviously" did not have working brake lights, thereby forcing his client to swerve to avoid rear-ending it. The jury deliberated all day. Finally they announced their decision after it had nearly become a hung jury.

It was a fair award but my law firm and I got only 60 percent of it. You see, the jury determined the driver of the car to be only 60 percent responsible for causing the accident. Amazingly, they held the large box of garbage in the road accountable for the other 40 percent. The lawyers representing me were flabbergasted. They couldn't believe the verdict. But I could. Only I—The Luckiest Unlucky Man Alive—could expect a box to leave me holding the bag.

As the one-year anniversary of my radical neck surgery approached, I started getting spiffed up, kind of like the Tin Man when he first visited Oz. First, Doc Sandler, head of the Ears, Nose and Throat Clinic and a real pro, did a Z-plasty on the long, thick, inflexible scar running down my neck. It was cut into and given two opposing wedge shaped cuts in the sign of the "Z," leaving me looking like I had lost a fight with Zorro. This was supposed to give the scar greater flexibility and movement and to blend it into the creases and folds of the neck—hopefully making the scar more cosmetically appealing. Well, it did make it more flexible. Also my dermatologist, Doc Schmieder excised a few questionable looking moles on my back that thankfully proved to be benign after the biopsy work was done.

When the cosmetically appealing aspect of the Z-plasty didn't work, a few months later Doc Sandler brought out a tool that worked like a Craftsman belt sander and dermabraided my scar down to the "Yuck!"

As the one year mark neared, the Navy hospital got their first plastic surgeon, Lieutenant Commander Eric Weiss. Young, cocky, and incredibly gifted in the latest cutting edge procedures of modern day plastic surgery, he played the part well. He also needed interesting cases to pass his Plastic Surgery Boards. I was deemed the perfect guinea pig.

Dr. Weiss insisted on doing the first ear reconstructive surgery under general anesthesia. It involved the painful removal of a four-inch piece of one of my ribs. This combination of bone and cartilage was then whittled down to size and inserted under the skin on the left side of my head. For a month, it was to be like an ear in a cocoon, waiting to bust loose and blow free in the wind like any other ear.

Just before I went under I told Doc Weiss, "Don't take any more rib than you need Eric. I know a lot of you surgeons have god complexes, but if you try to turn a piece of my rib into a woman, you'll be doing the whole world a terrible disservice."

"Why's that?" he smiled.

"Because she's gonna be UUGGLLEE! But, it gets worse. Her ego will be so huge that she'll never know how UUGGLLEE she really is!!!"

I was in the hospital for only a few days this time. One cute card I read while there waxed poetically:

"...*Thinking of you at this special time...and hoping your organ removal went fine....*"

The rib incision was unbelievably painful, as if Evander Holyfield had just hit me in the solar plexus with a sledgehammer. When I got home, I had a sealed test tube hanging from an incision behind my left ear. The test tube, half full of blood, was dangling from the side of my head like a Christmas ornament.

"You'd better not go outside, Daddy," Brian warned. "You'll be pecked to death by hummingbirds." As he said that, he pointed out the kitchen window to our hummingbird feeder dangling in the breeze and half full of red sugar water. It looked exactly like the test tube full of blood hanging from the left side of my head.

"Thanks, Brian." I retorted, "I guess that means you can empty the garbage."

During the month-long wait between my plastic surgeries, Dr. Weiss took his color *Encyclopedia of Reconstructive Surgery* off his shelf and showed me, in photographic detail, his plan of attack on my ear. He also showed me photos of children born with gaping cleft palates that stretched from the top to bottom of their faces. One poor little six-year-old Peruvian girl's face was so horrid I could not continue to look at the photograph. It made my disfigurement seem completely and totally insignificant.

"Now look at this," Doc Weiss stated matter-of-factly, as he held up a photograph of a beautiful sixteen-year-old girl.

"What's the point, Eric?" I asked as I looked at the pretty young woman.

"It's the same girl, ten years and 25 operations later. American doctors fly down to South America twice a year to volunteer their services. It's payback for our God-given talents."

I pictured Doc Weiss holding his hands to the heavens, with lightning striking all around and proclaiming, "These hands have been blessed by God!" And you know what? Like most good doctors and nurses, he would have been right.

I requested the remainder of my operations be done under local anesthesia. It was entertaining to listen to the lively banter between doctors and nurses as they forgot they had a "live one" on the table. For the next operation, Doc Weiss sliced the top of my ear free and then took a two-inch wide and six-inch long slice of skin from my left thigh. He then used it as a skin graft on the freshly opened skinless wound behind my ear.

A week later Doc Weiss looked at my ear and disappointedly stated, "Bill, this is bad. The whole graft and some of the cartilage is dead and nearly infected. We've got to start all over again first thing tomorrow morning."

"Oh, well," I figured, "...ear we go again...." But I was very disappointed. I knew where the next skin graft was coming from.

The next day, he took another nice-sized slice of flesh from my leg and an even thicker one from my groin, reworking the whole mess into something much less likely to reject the grafts.

He declared it a success a few weeks later. "You've got the start of a whole new ear again. No more need to grow long hair only on the left side of your head. But speaking of hair, the top of your left ear is now covered with your thigh and groin skin. So, you'll have to shave your ear everyday, or have electrolysis done on it at a hair removal salon. And also Bill—if your left ear gets warm when your pretty wife kisses you goodnight— I'm sure you'll be able to figure out why."

Our house on Fleming Island, near Jacksonville, Florida, was a veritable zoo. Peggy, and I wanted our twins, Brian and Christie, to develop the same love for nature and animals as we had when we were children. We've had tortoises and turtles, snakes, iguanas, frogs, rabbits, a three-pound attack Yorkie named "Scooter," young raccoons and even a wayward baby armadillo for a spell. But our lives were changed when Rocky came to stay.

When someone showed up at the local vet clinic with a tiny baby flying squirrel that had fallen from his nest, Dr. John Rossi reasoned that if a baby flying squirrel couldn't help a recovering cancer patient, nothing could. Dr. Rossi always had a knack for experimental therapies and must have figured "Why...well...why not...?" So he gave us Rocky to take home.

Rocky became an immediate fixture in the Goss household. When he first arrived, he was like a little ball of dust. He was the size of a walnut but weighed less. Rocky's eyes had just recently opened and he drank formula and water from a small toy baby bottle.

He'd barely move and his fur was kind of oily, like a greaser from the 50s. His bulging black eyes looked like aviator goggles, and Brian and Christie, having just seen an old cartoon rerun of "Rocky and Bullwinkle" named him.

He grew quickly and was soon about the size of a fresh bar of soap, his adult size. I say "his" with only minor skepticism, as Dr. Rossi had astutely stated during Rocky's gender evaluation, "Well, let's put him on a motorcycle and see if he sits on the front or the back."

Rocky's fur turned a silky smooth brown as he learned to clean himself regularly, and his eyes grew even more bulgy. His loose skin and his flat rudder-like tail turned him into a rodent frisbee during his daily flying lessons which I conducted by gently tossing him from our bathroom onto our bed. I figured I would initially know more about flying (they actually glide, not fly) than he did—but Rocky didn't require much training.

Flying squirrel movements are extremely fast and vertically oriented. Just like in the wild where they rapidly run up and down tree trunks, Rocky would run up and down our bodies, moving like a high scoring furred pinball on a flesh and blood pinball machine.

At the speed of light he is all over the inside and outside of our clothing as we try to catch him with our bare hands. The tickling, particularly when he dives into one of his favorite haunts, the armpits, is incredible, and is a daily ritual in our household, wonderfully lifting our spirits. If laughter is the best medicine, then Rocky delivered it by the truckload.

One morning I was enjoying my morning coffee like most people do, except that I had a newspaper in front of me and a squirrel on top of me. Rocky was sitting on my head surveying his squirreldom. Suddenly I sneezed. It was a big sneeze—one that occurred as I was bringing my cup to my lips. As I re-opened my eyes while continuing to bring my lukewarm coffee to my mouth, there were two of the most enormous, bulging eyes I'd ever come face-to-face with. It was a furred hyperthyroidic monster if I'd ever seen one. "Peggy, there's a flying squirrel in my coffee!" I yelled, laughing hysterically as my wife sprinted into the room. In an instant Rocky was back on my head preening himself, probably getting a caffeine buzz to boot.

I picked the newspaper back up, then quickly put it back down in a moment of reflection. I was overcome by a philosophical contemplation...that I am what I am, and that what I am is an utterly unique being—for, absolutely unquestionably—I was the only person in the world that had a flying squirrel in his coffee that morning.

Soon Rocky was sound asleep under my sweater, unaware of my earth-shattering musing, curled up on one of the large scars at the base of my neck.

Rocky—and God—were doing their healing magic once again.

Luckily we still have our pet flying squirrel Rocky to help keep our spirits high. Bill just adores having Rocky climb up and down his body like a tree trunk, only to fall fast asleep on the scars of his left shoulder. I love watching them play together. Animals—and that special brand of humor they bring to us—will always be a big, big part of our lives.

"The best way to know life is to live many things."
—Vincent Van Gogh

CHAPTER ELEVEN

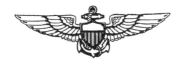

THE FIVE Fs OF FULFILLMENT AND THE HEALTHY HUMAN SPIRIT

"To laugh often and much;
to win the respect of intelligent people
and the affection of children;
to earn the appreciation of honest critics and
endure the betrayal of false friends;
to appreciate beauty; to find the best in others;
to leave the world a bit better whether by a healthy child;
a garden patch, or a redeemed social condition;
to know even one life has breathed easier because you have lived.
This is to have succeeded."
—Ralph Waldo Emerson

Although I had always planned to be able to retire before the age of forty, I quite honestly never could have imagined it would be under medical conditions for a highly malignant cancer. Yet still I count my blessings and they are many.

- I was blessed to be born an American, in a land of unbelievable freedoms and opportunities.
- I was blessed to be born into a two-parent home.
- I was blessed to have been given the opportunity to serve my country as a member of the military in the finest and most professional Armed Forces in the world.

- I was blessed to have been destined to form a union with a lasting and loving soulmate, thereby being able to experience the life-enriching joys of being a father and a husband.
- I was blessed with a cadre of stimulating lifelong friends each with a great sense of humor.
- I was blessed with a beautiful and healthy family.
- I was blessed with a focus on what's really important.
- I was blessed with a healthy human spirit.
- And I was blessed with enough adversities and challenges throughout my life to make me realize I'm *The Luckiest Unlucky Man Alive.*

People have often referred to me as lucky—because of all the things that have happened to me. Other people have often referred to me as unlucky—because of all the things that have happened to me. Someone once said that there is no such thing as luck, unless you call luck the product of unbridled determination and enthusiasm. Whoever that someone was I'd have to agree. It seems the profession one picks to make a living plays a big part in this "enthusiasm" equation. Ideally money should be the by-product of doing something you enjoy, not drudgery.

I chose to work on underwater bombs as an enlisted man, and later, I reached for the sky to become a commissioned officer and a Navy pilot. I didn't know how limited my abilities were at the time or I would have quit trying so hard a long time ago. Lucky for me, unlimited enthusiasm, perseverance, and my human spirit made me blind to my limited abilities, taking me to places where my intellectual and athletic abilities could never have led me.

What I've cherished my whole life, and what I'll reflect upon as I die after a brief illness at the age of 125, is not work, not money, not success, but on what I call the 5 Fs of Fulfillment: Family, Friends, Faith, Focus and Fun.

The came to me one day when I found myself staring at my left hand while getting a CAT scan. Why was I staring at my hand? Maybe because there is nothing else to stare at when flat on your back in a CAT scan machine. I was scared. My fingers were shaking. Suddenly as I spread my five fingers at arms length from my eyes, it dawned on me that maybe the meaning of life, at least my life, was right there in front of my face. WHAM! Like a fist between the eyes, suddenly those five fingers became the 5 Fs of Fulfillment: Family, Friends, Faith, Focus and Fun. Of course, Dr. Rat was quick to point out that if I had six fingers the sixth finger would just have to be for Fornication. But that's Rat for you, always thinking.... Forgiveness would fit.

The 5 Fs of Fulfillment are an ever-present reminder to me of what's important in life. I'll reflect on FAMILY: and on the endless love and support that Peggy provided the children and me through the years, throughout sickness and health, rain and shine. She's a terrific friend, lover and mother. A line from Jackson Browne's "I'm Alive" album sums up my feelings for Peggy:

> *"When I see the light upon her upturned face*
> *I can hear the angels sing...*
> *No one could ever take her place,*
> *I'll do anything...."*

I'll reflect on Brian and Christie, our two adorable children, who kept me laughing, loving, and proud as I learned about life the only real way possible, by helping children grow. I'll think about my mother and father who weren't perfect, but came as close as parents could get. And about brothers, and sisters, and aunts, and uncles, and grandparents, all of whom imprinted their smile on me at one time or another.

I'll reflect on FRIENDS: on old friends and new friends and friends yet to meet. And I'll think about lost opportunities—not in business, but in relationships—having learned that the bottom line shouldn't always be the top priority.

I'll reflect on FAITH: and about having faith even when nothing makes any sense at all. I'll think about the faith to believe that all those apostles couldn't have sided with the wrong guy.

I'll reflect on FOCUS: the power to know what is best for you. When to say, "No Sir" to your boss and "Yes Dear" to your wife and kids. By focusing on the other four Fs, energy is no longer scattered and diffused. The things you want done get done. Focus on the prize, whatever you choose that to be. Just make sure it's truly worthy of your time away from your family and friends.

And I'll reflect on FUN: the fun of enjoying animals and nature. The fun of special times with family and friends. The fun of being a husband and dad. The fun of sports and competition, the fun of flying and adventure. The fun of being an individual and being open-minded. The fun of going to the very limits of one's personal goals. The fun of laughing—the fun of just being alive.

Like the five fingers on your hand, the most valuable things in life are virtually free. Air, water, true friendship, freedom of thought, love, the ability to exercise both your mind and your body, the list goes on and on. It is typically the most meaningless things in life that cost us the most—cocaine, tobacco, alcohol, gratuitous entertainment, the latest, the greatest, the newest—the costs can be astounding—the returns devastating.

How do you get your life straightened out? How do you supercharge both your life and your immune system? Simple. Don't take the "free stuff" for granted. Live the 5Fs of Fulfillment each and every day like your life depends on them—because it does, at least the quality of your life does. This is what is takes to maintain a healthy human spirit.

What is demanded of humanity is not, as some existentialists believe, to endure the meaninglessness of life. Instead man should learn to accept his incapacity to understand unconditional meaningfulness in rational terms. In his acceptance, he will make something of himself—he will be self-determining. This concept is the basis for my belief in God, Faith and Humanity.

New research indicates that regret is one of our most powerful and complex emotions. Some say that we are so fearful of regret that we don't even want to talk about it, afraid that it will drag us down into a pit of depression and despair.

I say put your shortcomings out there for everyone to see. Be the first to laugh at them and watch your regrets melt away to become simply a part of your life, not the totality of your life. And remember, if you can find a path with no obstacles, no hardships, no challenges, no adversities—don't take it—it's a path that will lead you to nowhere.

You know, it seems to me that many people are searching for a reason to live. Well, I'm not. I figure I must be searching for a reason to die, because every time I've come close to death—except once—I decided consciously or subconsciously that death was the easy way out there is just too much to live for. And, like turning pages in a good book—I can't wait to see what the future chapters will bring.

There will come a juncture in all our
lives when its time to give up the fight
and set ourselves free from the confines and
limitations of our bodies.
Believe me, when that moment
arrives most of us will know it—
and it will be a blessing.
But for now, live your life,
enjoy your family and friends,
and put something positive into the world.
Enjoy your wild ride overcoming life's greatest challenges!

"When a man's eager and willing,
even the gods join in ...."
—Aeschlylus, Greek Dramatist

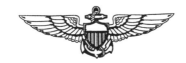

SUPERCHARGE YOUR IMMUNE SYSTEM NOW!

T he best way to survive cancer is to reduce your exposure to cancer risks. Smoking causes lung cancer, drinking excessively causes liver cancer and over-exposure to the sun causes skin cancer. It is a totally miserable disease. I can think of a hundred other diseases I'd rather have. Unfortunately, I had no choice.

If you are unable to prevent cancer, then the next best thing is to survive cancer. Early detection and aggressive treatment is the key. If something is not right, get it checked out right away. Persist until you get answers that are logical, not ones that please you. If your doctor isn't both a straight shooter and an optimist, get another doctor. Despite bad odds, some people recover from some pretty horrible stuff. Doctors sometimes forget that fact, even though it happens all around them, everyday.

Next, seek out rapid aggressive treatment. The choices were easy for me: scars and pain, or no scars and death. An easy choice for me.

Bizarre, difficult to diagnose forms of malignant melanoma like mine don't often pop up. Melanomas are usually much easier to diagnose than the little clear-skin bump that popped up on my ear. Typical melanomas, if detected early enough, usually involve simple surgery. But if you procrastinate, sometimes even for a day, the disease will become life threatening, the surgery and treatment very radical.

One theory about malignant cancer is that a *single* cancerous cell can multiply and spread throughout your body and kill you. According to other oncology theorists, this is true—but the chance that a single cancer cell can successfully fight your immune system, successfully multiply into a tumor and successfully spread to other parts of your body are a billion to one odds at any given moment.

These researchers argue that typical everyday folk have millions of cancer cells swimming among the trillions of normal healthy human tissue cells. They are constantly being gobbled up by a powerful immune system, even some of those cancer cells that have formed small microscopic tumors. Many researchers seem to agree that it is only when a tumor achieves a critical mass, a certain indeterminate number of cells, that it then becomes truly a threat to the host organism—you.

According to the 700-page, but easy-to-read book *Everyone's Guide to Cancer Therapy* by Dr. Malin Dollinger, (Somerville House), my little pea-sized tumor contained approximately one billion cancer cells. If you want to beat cancer, you must first understand it. The time-honored words of the warrior are "Know thy enemy." The first twenty pages of Dr. Dollinger's book superbly prepare you to be a smarter warrior in your fight against a tumor's doubling rate.

Obviously when the tumor gets too big, it overwhelms the billions of cells that comprise your immune system. This depends, of course, on how much you have strengthened your immune system and prepared it for battle.

I believe I boosted my immune system significantly by taking DHEA (dehydroepiandrosterone) as soon as I was diagnosed. I take DHEA every morning when I wake up. I believe it helped me in a large variety of unique ways. *The Superhormone Promise* by Dr. William Regelson (Simon & Schuster) discusses the remarkable characteristics of DHEA, a hormone that is produced by our adrenal glands in great abundance when we are twenty, much less when we are forty, and almost none at all when we are sixty.

I believe DHEA supplementation helped my deep scars melt away and has allowed me to do as many as ninety fingertip pushups in a row, even without a left trapezius muscle. I caution men, however, to take DHEA in the morning when they wake up. If they take it in the evenings, they may wake up with a "diamond-cutter" in the middle of the night. If they take it in the morning, they'll walk it off all day long.

And finally, one more extraordinary book about supercharging our immune system is *Your Body's Many Cries for Water*. This remarkable book by Dr. F. Batmanghelidj (*Global Health Solutions*, 703-848-2333) explains how so many health problems are directly related to chronic dehydration, often from caffeine. His credentials are so impeccable and his reasoning so sound that before you finish his book you will never again take for granted how important plenty of everyday tapwater is for supercharging your immune system.

Some researchers suggest that melanoma is not caused by the sun, but by flourescent lighting or other bizarre means. But most doctors agree the cancerous cells of malignant melanoma invade skin previously damaged by the sun's radiation, more often than not, during a bad childhood sunburn.

Biogenetic research is changing the entire field of cancer study. Within the past decade, oncogenes, genes that initiate the metastasis of cancer, have been found to exist within virtually all human organs. If we can find what sets off these oncogenes, then we should be able to find a way to stop cancer in its tracks. Researchers believe that when these genes are damaged—via smoking, environmental pollutants or intense radiation, even from the sun—cancer cells are set to explode within the weakened tissue.

Recently, researchers at the University of Colorado developed a form of gene therapy that appears to stop the spread of melanoma—which they describe as the fastest growing form of cancer within the human population. They hope it will not be too long before a melanoma vaccine genetically customized for the individual is available.

Malignant melanoma detected early is normally curable. However in a matter of weeks or months it can become deadly and spread throughout the lymphatic and circulatory systems to the brain, heart, lungs—anywhere—and everywhere. Ignoring a seemingly harmless mole or bump has put many, many people into an early grave.

Some families have genetic make-ups that put their skin—and lives—at risk. They are usually light skinned, blue-eyed, with blond, red or reddish brown hair. If you have a family history of melanoma and you fit the light skinned profile with moles, you should get examined by a dermatologist and plan a routine of follow-up examinations for the rest of your life. I am light skinned, blue-eyed, with light brown hair, though I was a towhead as a boy growing up. However, I don't have a lot of moles and my family had no prior history of melanoma.

You can improve your chances of not contracting melanoma by regularly looking at yourself naked in a full-length mirror. If you already feel sick at the thought of examining yourself this way, then you, my friend, are already in pretty bad shape—of course I'm only kidding. Carefully examine any moles, birthmarks or bumps, particularly in the more hidden parts of your body, like beneath your finger and toenails; on the soles of your feet and between your toes; in your scalp and under your arms; on your back and groin.

The National Cancer Institute suggests you think of A-B-C-D to help you figure out if a mole or birthmark is potentially deadly.

A is for Asymmetry—one side does not match the other.
B is for Border—the edges are ragged, ill defined.
C is for Color—the color is uneven, with various shading.
D is for Diameter—it is greater in diameter than the end of a pencil eraser.

If you have a birthmark or a mole (called a nevus by the skin docs) that fails one or more of the ABCD test—go see a dermatologist NOW. If you have a mole or birthmark that has changed in appearance, feel, or touch, particularly if it itches, bleeds or oozes—go see a dermatologist NOW. If you have a growing bump under your skin and it continues to increase in size each day—go see a dermatologist NOW.

Although malignant melanoma is less likely found in darker skinned people, it still develops on the less pigmented areas of their bodies, like the soles of the feet, palms of the hands and under finger and toe nails. It is critical that melanoma be detected very early before it penetrates deeper into the skin, tapping into a heavier blood supply, feeding the tumor and providing an easier route for it to spread via the bloodstream and lymphatic systems.

For your health's sake I must reiterate; the sooner a melanoma—or any tumor—is found, the easier the treatment. Act fast and aggressively if you think you are at risk and it will help to minimize the extent of any surgery you might soon require.

Amazingly, a dermatologist at the Tallahassee Medical Center has trained George, a schnauzer, to sniff out potentially deadly melanomas on the surfaces of human skin. Like a bloodhound on the scent of a killer, George can detect the incredibly small differences in odor concentrations, concentrations more minute than even one part per billion. I sure wish George had been around to sniff my ear before my melanoma had turned into an obvious lump. But with my luck—like Garp's—or Evander Holyfield's—George the dog would have bitten my left ear off.

Cancer is regarded by some as holding the key to the fountain of youth, because where normal tissue cells can multiply 50 to 100 times before they weaken and die, cancer cells can apparently live and multiply forever. It's possible that the same researchers who discovered how cancer cells multiply and live forever will also uncover the secret of how to prevent normal cells from aging and dying, discovering a kind of cellular fountain of youth. So far, no one's survived life. That may change in the future. What would we do with everybody?

One melanoma survivor, Shaun Hughes, created a company called Sun Precautions, Inc. which manufactures cool and lightweight protective clothing for particularly sun sensitive people and for those who spend a lot of time outdoors. His company appears to be thriving as people become more and more aware of the dangers from sun overexposure. Shaun turned his "bad" experience into a beneficial and profitable company. He epitomizes the natural entrepreneurship that is the key to surviving cancer—the ability, even the spirit—to turn something bad into something good. A positive spirit must have a favorable effect on the immune system compared to the effect that negative or "downer" inputs would have on the autonomic systems of the body.

If someday a form of malignant cancer is found in your body (the odds are greater than 50 percent that this will happen) spend some time in despair, and then get over it. Author and Yale Surgeon Dr. Bernie Siegel offers tremendous insights in his book *Love, Medicine and Miracles* (Harper and Row) on how to speed your recovery by combining natural healing techniques with sound medical practices. He claims that medical treatment is only as effective as the patient's unconscious thoughts allow it to be. Furthermore, only a combination of stress reduction, conflict resolution, visualization and positive reinforcement can stimulate the immune system and allow healing to take place. He says that for a lot of people, "generally...cancer is an easy way out."

One of the first questions he asks his patients is, "Do you want to live to be one hundred?" If the answer is a genuine yes, he knows he has an exceptional patient in his care, one capable of self-induced healing.

He believes that learning to let go of negative emotions is pivotal to the healing process. A bad attitude slows down all the vital "live" mechanisms, the immune globulins, endorphins, white blood cells and other internal healing components of the body.

To break down the "I'm in control, I'll determine whether you are going to live or die" doctor/patient barrier, Dr. Siegel insists his patients call him by his first name. Bernie also tells them, "If you want to die, stay depressed; if you want to live, then love and laugh." Positive emotions stimulate the immune system. People who share and talk with their physicians—and who choose their therapies for positive reasons—have maybe one-fourth to one-tenth the side effects of people who just silently submit to treatment because their doctors or spouses insisted upon it.

Studies have shown that patients who physicians say are their biggest pests are actually the ones whose immune systems are the most active. They are the long-term survivors. The most important contribution a doctor can make is to give the patient control over his or her treatment. The second is to offer hope. There's no such thing as false hope. Hope is real and physiological.

Dr. Siegel states "The best advice I can give to anybody is to live each day as if it were your last. I'm talking from a spiritual standpoint. Make yourself happy. Resolve your conflicts. Get things off your chest. Find that peace of mind, that clear conscience. I'll guarantee you'll wake up the next morning feeling so good, you won't want to die."

The National Cancer Institute, quoting what Bernie would call an "exceptional patient," published,

> "Cancer survivorship can be a catalyst for spiritual awakening, providing life with depth and poignancy...developed with utmost clarity, while superficial distractions and frivolous people are filtered out...[Survivors] share a new understanding of time, a sense of needing to make every minute count."

That certainly has been my experience. There is so much I want to accomplish that I don't think even living to be 125 will provide me with enough time to get it all done. Freud once said, "the older one grows the more there is to do." The more experiences a person has the wiser they should be—and the more they can give others.

I believe we must foster a fire within ourselves, an anima, like a super spirited animal, like a jaguar on the jungle floor or a goshawk maneuvering at high speed through the tightly spaced trees of a virgin redwood forest. Whether wrestling on the ground or in the air, the indomitable and raw tenacity of these two animals have always held great meaning for me. But, as long as I'm on this earth, I'm sure it's the jaguar in me that will keep me fighting and keep my spirit burning well past 2080, the year I turn 125 years old.

During my first surgery, many nerves were severed on the left side of my face and neck, causing a loss of control to the muscle and skin tension of my throat. When I fell asleep my windpipe would collapse and the snoring and sleep apnea was so severe that Peggy, Brian and Christie, and even the guys on the five day whitewater rafting trip all threatened to abandon me.

Dr. Mark Frey performed laser surgery on my throat to help end my bouts with dangerous sleep apnea by enlarging the tiny hole I had once called a windpipe. As the laser cooked my throat, I smelled the incredible stink—and could taste—my own flesh frying. But at least it was my flesh. You know the old adage, "When it comes from yourself you can stand it."

To kill the pain during the surgery I put myself into a self-hypnotic trance. I dreamed I was a hawk flying along a heavily treed mountain ridge surveying my domain and studying the ground for prey. I was a goshawk, the most tenacious and fearless flyer of the deep forest, the raptor of choice among kings and nobility. It was while self-hypnotically transposed into that powerful and proud bird of prey, that I first envisioned my logo for GOSHAWK INTERNATIONAL, a company I started using my old nickname.

People, and especially pilots, imagine personal disaster as something that only falls on the other guy. Call it dreams of invulnerability or call it stupidity, sooner or later the real world smashes flat their house of cards with a challenge of immense proportions.

As a guy who routinely partook in dangerous endeavors, I always tried to provide myself "with a way out" before going into a sticky situation. Maybe it was simply "street smarts" I learned from my experiences with the Gabers. But whatever it was, when I wasn't able to "leave myself an out" I always ended up praying like hell. Some of these things required instant response but many required much thought and contemplation.

Each person has his or her own unique way of dealing with such things. Mine is to take stock in all the things I hold near and dear to me, things I have nurtured throughout my life. I would reflect on other times when ugly challenges have turned into personal redemptions and devastating family crisis into thankful and enduring family memories. In times like these we prove to be far tougher and more durable than we could ever imagine ourselves to be.

I am reminded of a friend and neighbor who helped me during my recovery. Pat Coyle, whose mother died of cancer, mowed our lawn during the period of time I was drugged and bedridden after my cancer surgery. During Navy flight training, Pat had ejected from an A-4 Skyhawk jet as it moved uncontrollably toward the edge of the runway during his takeoff roll. As he floated down in his parachute he saw a jet takeoff from the end of the runway. "I wonder whose jet that could be?" he said to himself. Moments later he realized his jet had taken off without him. Like an unmanned missile, the jet flew into a hangar, destroying twenty planes and killing a civilian maintenance man.

Devastated, Pat never got his Navy Wings of Gold, but he pressed on and became a Navy Aircraft Maintenance Officer, then a helicopter pilot in the U.S. Army Reserves. He now serves as a U.S. Customs pilot flying the Blackhawk helicopter in drug surveillance missions across the country. Pat lives down the river from me and we sometimes fly his 50-year-old seaplane together, landing on the local waterways. Pat pressed on with his dream of becoming a professional aviator when most people would have quit. He demonstrated the fortitude of his personal human spirit by never giving up on his dream.

While convalescing at home, in between a steady diet of bone scans, laboratory work-ups, CAT scans, lymph node palpations, chest X-rays and numerous reconstructive surgeries, I had some more time to think about what I was going to do over the next 85 or more years that I expect to live. I even told Doc Marsland when I first met him, "I'm looking for an oncologist that I know I'll outlive." Against those odds, he still took me on as a patient!

I figured that as a recovering cancer patient, I would be viewed as a poor risk for future employment, unhireable by the airlines and other industries because of Workman's Compensation liabilities. Yet I knew I would have to quickly formulate a plan to keep my mind going after retirement to help stave off depression. I also realized that moving up in a bureaucracy was no longer a pursuit that I desired in my life. I decided I would never again work for someone else simply to attain more power and more money.

While a Navy pilot, I received some support and encouragement from more senior officers in regards to my writing ability. Although several of my articles and proposals had been published or had made their way up the chain of command for review, the writing always had to be technical. The potential for getting innovative or humorous submissions accepted was all but eliminated. Official writing has to be, well you know, official. A famous comedian/writer/director who took a liking more to his stepdaughter than his wife once quipped that he had fulfilled all the prerequisite life experiences to be a successful writer. "...I've been a boxer, a sailor, a miner, a pilot...."

Well, I figured, that crack was meant as a joke, but I have been all those things...maybe I should become a full-time writer. And with the initials WAG, why shouldn't I be amusing as well?

After the car accident and the accompanying "out-of-body" experience, I found that the logical left-brained life I had led was being overcome by imaginative right-brained thinking. It seemed like I lost the capacity to function very well with highly technical things.

My mind instead sought to be more creative and expansive. It was almost as if my heart's desire had suddenly done a complete reversal in midstream. I began to enjoy creating rather than formulating, and modifying, rather than beating, deadlines. Although I still enjoyed competition, I could no longer take it seriously. I realized that life is too short for "one-upsmanship." This new way of looking at things was not at all disconcerting but instead gave me great pleasure as I began to evolve into a new me.

Having the opportunity to be creative, after an exciting, but not so creative career in underwater weapons and aviation, has been both refreshing, stimulating, and life affirming. Over the years and with advice and encouragement from friends, particularly Vicki Smith, Toysan Reed, Sarah Bewley and Janice Phelps, I began to write down my ideas and experiences.

I also started marketing several inventions I've created, with my brother Larry, Rat and Mark Ruberg, a fourth generation toolmaker and Ohio wrestling champion. We are seeking patent approval on one particular invention, a unique, three-dimensional leveling device which will hopefully be acquired by a major tool manufacturer. Our hero is Thomas Edison, a guy who just never learned the words "I quit," even after he tried over 2000 different materials in which to conduct electricity in a vacuum. He finally hit upon one, carbonized bamboo—and invented what we now know as the light bulb.

I travel out to Arizona to spend time with my old buddy

Steve Kauffman. Steve's a promising novelist and the President of Tucson Professional Trainers, the largest fitness training company in Tucson. He and his beautiful wife Normie live with their five wolves and extensive monitor lizard collection on John Wayne's former ranch in the foothills of the Sonoran Desert. We are now collaborating on several writing projects.

I joined the Florida Falconry Association and started going to falconry meets to learn more about hawking and the Goshawk specifically. I watched a goshawk fly in aerial combat against mallard ducks. What a regal and awe-inspiring bird of prey, completely alert and totally in command of the earth beneath his wings at over 100 miles per hour.

Peg, the kids and I adopted a wild goshawk that had been banded by the non-profit organization HawkWatch International so researchers could track it as it flew across America during its annual migration.

I was selected as an extra in *G.I. JANE*, a Demi Moore movie in which I played a naval officer. Demi bought me, and a lot of other people, dinner a few nights later, just after she shaved her head to the bone. She and I discovered we had a mutual friend in Rio de Janeiro, Caetano, a professional driver.

Two evenings a month I teach self-defense at the Quigley House and the Hubbard House, shelters for battered women with children. The bruises, cigarette burns and other physical scars on so many of these women are an obvious testimony to the hidden violence that they endure at the hands of their "loved ones." These shelters protect and hide women and their children during an extremely dangerous time—when they finally decide to leave their batterers.

One other thing Peg and I did during this period of personal redevelopment was to buy a very rustic wilderness cabin on a lake smack dab in the middle of Osceola National Forest. Like the Porsche, it was another wonderful bargain aided by my earlier earlessness. Surrounded by dense forest, it is the wilderness release site of the endangered Florida panther.

Tracked by radio telemetry by wildlife biologists, these panthers have been routinely spotted on or near our property since the beginning of the panther release program. Along with the Florida panther, we have diamondback, canebrake and pygmy rattlesnakes, cottonmouth water moccasins, coral snakes, wild boar, black bear, 14-foot gators and 18-pound largemouth bass. For me, it's like reliving the "Hotel" and "The Lake" experiences of my youth. It is wild and private and beautiful—and we love it.

One of my friends, Rudy Ruettiger, is tremendously inspirational to me. He's the guy who turned his own remarkable story about a small, dyslexic boy with a dream of playing football at Notre Dame into the wonderful TriStar blockbuster movie *RUDY*. If you haven't seen his movie, go to the video store and rent it. By the way, the *real* Rudy is as nice a person as he was depicted on the silver screen by actor Sean Astin, another great guy. Rudy is showing the screenplay adaptation of this book to Hollywood producers.

Having more time to spend with my family and friends and having the freedom to help local organizations like the Quigley and Hubbard Houses, has made me feel like I've been given a new lease on life. God knows that after all I've been through, I needed a new one.

So, like a flunky alchemist turning manure into shine-ola, I am turning my misadventures into a special form of personal empowerment. Writing, inspirational speaking, and inventing are what I now do for a living. I've always believed that when one door closes, another door opens. I hope you do too.

> *"May the road rise up to meet you.*
> *May the wind be always at your back,*
> *May the sun shine warm upon your face,*
> *The rains fall soft upon your fields,*
> *And until we meet again...*
> *May God hold you in the palm of his hand."*
> *—An Irish blessing read at Pop's memorial service*

"He who has the last laugh wins."
—The Gabers

INDEX OF CHARACTERS
OR GABERS, ET AL.

"Perseverance is not a long race,
it is many short races one after the other."
—Walter Elliot

People have expressed curiosity in what the future held for my boyhood friends. Peer pressure being the incredibly powerful motivator that it is—the Gabers and my other buddies persevered and became accomplished in a myriad of diverse professions. What is most remarkable is that none of us copied, duplicated or imitated career paths, or even chose to work with one another. With so much in common we all still found our own unique little niche in the world to lay claim to.

"Bloomer" aka David Bloom—Ivy League superachiever. Now a commercial real estate tycoon, Dave conceived a little interstate highway phenomenon—upscale factory outlet malls.

"Wildman Crowley" aka Richard Crowley—After a college partying career that will go down in the "University of Vermont's Annals of Infamy", he became a pilot and building contractor.

"Maid Marian" aka Marian Falla—Master's Degree in Marine and Environmental Science. Executive in an international gaming conglomerate.

"Snakeman" aka Douglas Finnegan—President and Founder of Insight Designs, a San Francisco based company.

"Grazzoo" aka Dave Graziano—An All-American Scholar-Athlete and later Harvard MBA, now in private business.

"Grimmer" aka John Grimm—Successful Wall Street Broker.

"Gureenie" aka Dr. Carl Guarino—Broard certified in both Ear, Nose and Throat Surgery and Radiology in northern New Jersey. Dr. Guarino was an essential source of information during my malignant melanoma-on-the-ear crisis.

"Jay Bird" aka John Hanson—Delta Airline pilot based out of Atlanta, Georgia.

"Derry" aka Derry Riddle Hogan—Accomplished commercial artist living in New Hampshire with her husband and two sons.

"Steve" aka Steve Kauffman—President and founder of Tucson Professional Trainers and an accomplished novelist.

"Killer" aka Jon Kilik—One of the top movie producers in the world, collaborating with the likes of Robert Dinero, Spike Lee and Tim Robbins to produce Academy Award winning movies like *Dead Man Walking*.

"Fuzz" aka Mark Landis—Master's Degree in Landscape Architecture. Landscape Director of historical sites at Jekyl Island, Georgia. Former All-American in the steeplechase who ran a 2:22 minute marathon.

"Boobus" aka Jeff Marcketta—After years working in his family's paint store, he earned a CPA. Presently serves as the Executive Vice President of Panavision International in Los Angeles. Our twins, Brian and Christie, call him "Uncle Beastie."

"Jungle James" aka Jim Mardis—After we bought some cheap lakefront property for no money down while in college, he turned this extremely profitable venture into one of the most successful real estate companies in New Hampshire.

"Brian Mee" aka Brian Mee—After getting out of the U.S. Navy, he earned a Master's Degree in Civil Engineering. He builds bridges and skyscrapers in Atlanta.

"Chelsea" aka Mike McCullough—President of a multi-million dollar manufacturing and sales company in Rhode Island.

"Cubie" aka Chris McHugh—Former N.J. State Champion pole-vaulter, he became an All-American runner at Penn State. As President of T.A. McHugh Company in New Jersey, he represents manufacturers in petrochemical and metal fabrication industries.

"Duvalle" aka Dennis McHugh—Still eternally "Duvalle." Some things never change.

"Bo" aka Pat Mills—Triathelete and future commanding officer of Patrol Squadron 45. One of the U.S. Navy's superstars.

"Stench ala Foof" aka Dr. Sandy North—Podiatrist in Miami, Florida. Ranked third in the United States in the men's open division for judo.

"Mo" aka Marty O'Hare—Owns and trains thoroughbred horses on a farm in South Jersey.

"Dr. Rat" aka Greg O'Neil—Founder and President of APEX Technologies. Designs and manufactures environmental sampling computer equipment. A licensed private pilot. Don't go flying when he's in the air. Funnier than ever.

"Harv" aka Harvey Perkins—Another friend of mine who became a private pilot, he is an executive at Showboat International Casinos, Atlantic City.

"Larry" aka Lawrence Rayko—After working in the underground mines with me, he graduated from the University of Arizona and disappeared into the mountains of Tibet, never to be heard from again. His picture should be on the back of milk cartons.

"Dan 'The Man' " aka Daniel Stouder—Restauranteur in Southern California.

"Stiff" aka Bob Vogt—Stockbroker in New Jersey. Nearly coaching his team to the World Series, the Gabers consider him the George Steinbrenner of Little League Baseball.

"Alice" aka Alice Chrystie Wyman—Worked in Manhattan as an editor and earned a Master's Degree in Education. Lives in New England with her husband, Peter, son of the former CEO of CBS, with their three sons.

"It has done me good
to be somewhat parched by the sun
and drenched by the rain of life."
—Longfellow